Contents

Evaluating Mental Health Services for Older People

Jenny Finch

**Foreword by
Bob Woods**

RADCLIFFE PUBLISHING
OXFORD · SAN FRANCISCO

Radcliffe Publishing Ltd
18 Marcham Road
Abingdon
Oxon OX14 1AA
United Kingdom

www.radcliffe-oxford.com
Electronic catalogue and worldwide online ordering facility.

British Library Cataloguing in Publication Data

A catalogue record for this book is available from the British Library.

ISBN 1 85775 610 X

Typeset by Acorn Bookwork Ltd, Salisbury
Printed and bound by TJ International Ltd, Padstow, Cornwall

Foreword

Mental health services for older people have come a long way in the last 40 years. No longer is it thought acceptable for older people with dementia and other mental health problems to be confined in Victorian lunatic asylums, well away from their community, with 'warehousing' and 'custodial care' being apt descriptors of their treatment. Many factors have led to this change, not least a general increase in societal expectations of care provided to vulnerable people. There have been great advances in our understanding of mental health problems across the life span and, especially in the UK, the pioneers of old age psychiatry led the way in developing service models based on providing a comprehensive service to a specified catchment area. Such services emphasised the importance of careful assessment, covering mental and physical health and social circumstances, of using available treatments and of building networks of care within the community. Increasingly, these services became multi-disciplinary, culminating in the development of community mental health teams for older people.

However, despite much progress, there is still great scope for improvement. In the UK, two major inquiries conducted by the Commission for Health Improvement concerned the quality of health services for older people with mental health problems. Mental health services for older people consistently fall between two stools when services are planned and resources allocated. The dilemma has long been whether it is better to be allied to mental health services 'for people of working age' or whether links to older people's services are more fruitful. Thus in England the National Service Framework for Older People includes a chapter on mental health, whilst there is a separate complete Framework devoted to mental health problems in younger adults. This difficulty reflects the intrinsic complexity of this area, where physical and mental health interact, where the effects of ageing and disease are interwoven, where the societal influences of ageism and stigma still operate, where family care continues to provide the bulk of the support despite the changing and dynamic nature of family structures.

A variety of service systems and sub-systems add to the complexity. Is the provision of day time support for a person with dementia a social care or a healthcare responsibility? When do physical problems dictate that the person with severe dementia should be looked after by a physician in geriatric medicine rather than an old age psychiatrist? Does a person who has been under the care of an adult mental health service for 40 years with recurrent episodes of psychotic depression need to be transferred to an old age psychiatrist on their 65th birthday? When resources are limited, it is inevitable that each sub-system will withdraw from generous collaboration and cooperation, and will focus only on those people meeting their eligibility criteria. Just as inevitably, some people will fall between services, and at worst be shuttled backwards and forwards between them, with each preserving its own territory, and no-one taking responsibility for the unfortunate patient caught in the middle.

When service evaluation is considered, it is tempting to examine immediately 'the evidence base', in the sense of the research literature examining the outcomes produced by the service. In fact, there are very few rigorous, controlled evaluations of different types of service approaches in this field. Even if there were, results obtained under the 'laboratory' conditions of a randomised controlled trial might not generalise to the real world of unselected patients, under-resourced staff and high case loads. As well as considering outcomes, we need to also look carefully at the process of service provision and the structures and other inputs that support these processes. Many concerned and committed practitioners in this field find themselves, in the rare moments they have for reflection, asking 'How are we doing? What difference are we making? How do we compare with other services? How do we develop the service for the benefit of service users? How could we operate more effectively?'

The service standards which Jenny Finch developed in her work with the Health Advisory Service were intended to be used in visits to services by peer reviewers – people who knew about service provision either by experience as a professional in such a service, or as a carer or user at the receiving end of such a service. Each review using these standards aimed to hold a mirror up to the service, to encourage reflection, self-assessment and action planning. It encouraged partnerships and joint working across systems by reflecting on the totality of the experience of the service user and carers. Each standard was based on the best available evidence and policy guidance, and in this book Jenny has presented an approach to considering the validity and reliability of these standards. This does suggest that the standards-based approach is indeed a significant step forward from the previous pattern of the review team applying their own implicit yardstick.

This endeavour raises fascinating questions regarding the most effective strategy for driving forward the quality of services. In contrast to the reflective approach adopted by the Health Advisory Service in the late 1990s, Jenny also writes with experience of the more inspectorial approach of the then Commission for Health Improvement. Armed with more teeth, but perhaps a slightly more broad brush approach, it is interesting to speculate whether this had more impact. In each case, clear action plans with agreed targets were seen as essential to monitor the process of change, but it could be argued that an approach which fully engaged and involved practitioners would be crucial if the experience of service users were to be changed.

The problem is often simply where to start. Services are multicomponent, multilevel, multidisciplinary, with so many layers of complexity, that a key part of any evaluation is to assist in decisions about the priority of possible actions and improvements, balancing what is achievable with what will make most impact. Jenny's international perspective in this book serves as a useful reminder that there is usually more than one way of achieving a goal and that, although in any one country there may be many changes of policies and structures, the essentials remain: a focus on a person-centred approach, a need for coordination of service response, the adoption of multidisciplinary working and a commitment to continuous quality improvement. There are now a range of agencies and individuals who are charged with or have a commitment to taking forward services for older people with mental health problems. In this book, Jenny Finch offers an invaluable starting point to understanding the historical and international context of such services, and provides a good basis for considering evaluation systems aiming to contribute to quality improvement.

Bob Woods
Professor of Clinical Psychology of Older People
University of Wales Bangor
June 2004

Preface

There is broad recognition that, despite some examples of promising practice, there is a need for improvements overall in services for older people with mental health problems in the United Kingdom (UK). Research (Audit Commission 2000, 2002; Department of Health 2003b) has found that services were patchy and inconsistent across the country. Mental health services for older people emerged as a specialty area in the UK from the 1960s, and Chapter 1 traces that development. Because of the complexity of their needs, older people with mental health problems are one of the service user groups for which, it is said, an integrated approach in service planning and provision is particularly important. Chapter 2 therefore provides an account of the policy background to such an integrated approach in relation to this group, and the scope for successful integration is considered.

The development of old age psychiatry as a discipline internationally, in the 1980s and 1990s, followed that in the UK. However, the creation of a range of services specifically to meet the needs of older people with mental health problems has been variable in some parts of the world. While there are models of promising practice in planning and provision of services, countries may have concentrated on certain types of service at the expense of others, or their focus on dementia, while important, may have meant that older people with other sorts of mental illness have received less attention. Services for older people with mental health problems in Europe, the United States of America (USA), Canada and Australia are discussed in Chapters 3 to 15.

To see evaluation of mental health services for older people in context, some consideration is required of the various approaches to evaluating health and social care, and this is provided in Chapters 16 to 19. The models discussed include accreditation, the European Foundation for Quality Management and other mechanisms used in Europe, and the countries considered are, again, the UK, Europe, the USA, Canada and Australia. With regard to the UK, the main government-led systems for assessing health and social care services are discussed in Chapter 20, including the Commission for Health Improvement, the Social Services Inspectorate and their companion organisations (several of which became part of the Healthcare Commission or the Commission for Social Care Inspection in 2004).

From 1997 to 2000, the (then) Health Advisory Service (HAS) undertook a programme to develop standards and methodologies to evaluate services for its client groups, including mental health services for older people. The approach comprised systematic mechanisms for identification of relevant publications, content analysis and consultation with professionals, users and carers to produce the standards, and use of an evidence base and consultation in devising the methodology. Aspects of this approach were designed to ensure the standards' validity, and research was undertaken to test that validity and the standards' reliability in use.

Chapters 23 and 24 provide an account of the methodology used in devising the HAS standards, and Chapters 25 to 27 describe how their validity and reliability were tested. The results of the reliability test produced useful findings, with regard to the creation of robust standards and ensuring consistency in the methods used in applying them, that is to say, in service reviews. These are discussed in Chapter 29.

Jenny Finch
June 2004

About the author

Jenny Finch worked for several years in joint health and social care policy in Lewisham and Croydon, where she had a major role in devising and implementing strategies on inequalities and health, health promotion and community care. She then moved to evaluation of health and social care at a national level. At the Health Advisory Service (HAS), she led the development of standards and methodologies, and managed reviews, to evaluate mental health services for older people, and child and adolescent mental health services. She edited the HAS series of standards for all its client groups. At the Commission for Health Improvement she led the development of the methodology for reviewing clinical governance in health authorities and primary care.

Jenny then worked in the Department for Education and Skills in the Children's Fund Team, and then as team leader on disability and inclusion in the Sure Start Unit, before moving to her post as Children and Young People's Strategic Partnership Manager in Islington. She previously carried out much community development work on health issues, in particular with women and older people.

Jenny is also a linguist in French and Italian, and a qualified translator.

ACKNOWLEDGEMENTS

I would like to thank Martin Orrell and Ann Bowling for their advice on methodological issues. I am grateful to Paul Lelliott and Geoff Shepherd for their contribution to the development of standards and methodologies for service reviews, Alison Pearce for her contribution to devising the system of content analysis, and Charles Shaw for his advice on mechanisms for evaluating healthcare internationally. I would also like to thank Graham Dunn for his advice on methodology for testing reliability, and Barry Tennison and Gerrard Abi-Aad for their contribution on statistical data issues. My thanks to my family for their support throughout this project.

Abbreviations

AAA	Area Agency on Aging
ABHB	Alberta Mental Health Board
ACHS	Australian Council on Health Care Standards
ADM	alcohol, drug abuse and mental health
ALPHA	Agenda for Leadership in Programs for Healthcare Accreditation
AIM	Achieving Improved Measurement (Program)
AMA	Australian Medical Association
CADE	confused and disturbed elderly
CCHSA	Canadian Council on Health Services Accreditation
CHAI	Commission for Healthcare Audit and Inspection
CHAP	Community Health Accreditation Program
CHI	Commission for Health Improvement
CMHC	Community Mental Health Center
CMHSD	Centre for Mental Health Services Development
CNAVTS	Caisse nationale assurance vieillesse travailleurs salariés
CPA	Care Programme Approach
CPA	comprehensive performance assessment
CPA	Centre for Policy on Ageing
DRG	diagnostic related groups
EFQM	European Foundation for Quality Management
ExPeRT	external peer review techniques project
GAT	geriatric assessment team
GMS	General Medical Services
GP	general practitioner
G theory	generalisability theory
HACC	Home and Community Care (Program)
HAP	Hospital Accreditation Programme
HAS	Health Advisory Service
HASCAS	Health and Social Care Advisory Service
HMO	health maintenance organisation
HQS	Health Quality Service
IPA	International Psychogeriatric Association
ISO	International Organization for Standardization
ISQua	International Society for Quality in Health Care
JCAHO	Joint Commission on Accreditation of Healthcare Organizations
KFOA	King's Fund Organisational Audit
MAPAD	Maisons d'accueil pour personnes âgées dépendantes
MHSFOP	mental health services for older people
NAPDC	National Action Plan for Dementia Care
NCSC	National Care Standards Commission

NICE	National Institute for Clinical Excellence
NSF	National Service Framework
NSW	New South Wales
OBRA	Omnibus Budget Reconciliation Act
OFSTED	Office for Standards in Education
PAF	performance assessment framework
PCG	primary care group
PCT	primary care trust
PSA	public service agreement
PSIGE	psychologists' special interest group – elderly
SD	standard deviation
SDA	service development adviser
SSI	Supplemental Security Income
SSI	Social Services Inspectorate
TRG	technical reference group
UK	United Kingdom
USA	United States of America
VA	Veterans' Affairs
WHO	World Health Organization
WPA	World Psychiatric Association

PART I

MENTAL HEALTH SERVICES FOR OLDER PEOPLE IN THE UNITED KINGDOM

CHAPTER 1

Development of services

Introduction

In this chapter, the development of mental health services for older people in the United Kingdom (UK) since the 1960s is traced. During this period, interest in these services has increased, partly in response to the growing number of older people, and a specialty has been created. The pressure on health and social services of the sheer numbers of old people, and the ageing of the elderly population itself contributed to the debate on the need for special services for older people who were psychiatrically ill (Arie and Isaacs 1978). In the 1970s and early 1980s, widespread acceptance emerged in Britain of the principle that there should be special psychiatric services for older people in each locality. This was also encouraged by the developments in psychiatry which made available effective biological, psychological, and organisational techniques which were of great relevance for older people, although older people were generally heavily under-represented as beneficiaries of these developments. Finally, the acceptance in the preceding decades that health services should be planned for defined populations had relevance to the establishment of district services for older people with mental disorders (Arie and Jolley 1982). Progress was such that in 1998, the Royal College of Psychiatrists and the Royal College of Physicians recommended that, by 2002, every health district should have a comprehensive, specialised service for the psychiatry of old age (Royal College of Psychiatrists and Royal College of Physicians 1998).

Components of mental health services for older people

In order to illustrate constant features and changes in emphasis in mental health services for older people over the past four decades, mention of certain key activities of these services in selected publications is included in Table 1.1. Community care/ outreach, outpatient facilities, day hospitals, day centres, and long-term hospital care have been among the constant features of services provided, or considered necessary. Emphasis on assessment units appears to have commenced in the early 1970s, and remained since then. The focus on respite care and support for carers as part of services appears to have emerged in the early 1990s, although the importance of such support was recognised earlier. This may reflect the requirements of the government's legislation and guidance on community care in the late 1980s and 1990.

The same legislation and guidance, with its emphasis on joint working, was likely to have been a motivation in the examination of the roles of other disciplines and agencies at this time; however, interest in this was also evident in the late 1970s. It seems to be at this stage that psychologists were starting to use techniques aimed specifically at older people. Clinical psychologists, who were only minimally involved with testing, began to explore the scope for behavioural modification techniques and psychotherapy with older people, and to conduct groups for patients and for relatives (Arie and Isaacs 1978).

Table 1.1: Mention of certain key activities of mental health services for older people in selected publications, 1960–98

	Macmillan 1960	Donovan et al. 1971	Arie and Isaacs 1978	Jolley and Arie 1992	RCPsych/ RCP* 1998
Community care/outreach	✓		✓	✓	✓
Outpatient facilities	✓		✓		✓
Assessment unit		✓		✓	✓
Joint psychiatric/ geriatric beds			✓		
Day hospital	✓	✓	✓		✓
Day centre	✓			✓	✓
Long-term hospital care	✓	✓			✓
Specialist residential homes	✓	✓			
Respite care				✓	✓
Support for carers				✓	
Work with other disciplines/ agencies			✓		✓
Advice/liaison				✓	✓
Education				✓	✓
Research				✓	✓

* Royal College of Psychiatrists and Royal College of Physicians.

Advice and liaison, education, and research, all emerged as features of these specific services in the 1990s. This was perhaps because, by that time, mental health services for older people had become sufficiently established as a specialty to undertake these functions.

The acceptance by the 1970s and 1980s of the need for special psychiatric services for older people is borne out in the increasing number of components of such services, which, using the categories selected for this exercise, rose from four to six in the 1960–78 period, to eight in 1992, and 11 in 1998.

Principles of mental health services for older people

Principles of mental health services for older people have included, as constant features, a comprehensive service for a defined population, treating the full range of mental disorders in older people, and availability and flexibility. Added to these, in the late 1970s, were principles that mirror the components of services described in the previous section: the ability to work with other disciplines, and, in the early 1990s, attention to the needs of caregivers, both professional and informal (Jolley and Arie 1978; Shulman and Arie 1991).

Development of posts of old age psychiatrist

In line with the general acceptance, from the late 1960s to the late 1970s, of the need in each health district for some differentiation of mental health services specifically for older people, posts of consultant psychiatrist 'with a special interest in the elderly' were, by the late 1970s, among the most commonly advertised posts in psychiatry. At the end of the 1960s there were less than six psychiatrists for whom this was their special interest; at the end of 1980, 120 consultant psychiatrists had psychiatry of old age as their main activity (10% of all consultant psychiatrists in the NHS). By 1986, some 250 consultants were providing specialised psychiatry services for nearly 70% of the elderly population of the UK, and a survey in 1993 identified 405 consultants working with populations ranging from 9000 to 40 000 older people (Jolley and Arie 1978; Arie 1989; Arie and Jolley 1982, 1998). A further survey carried out in 2001 identified a total of 553 clinically active old age consultant psychiatrists in England, Scotland, Wales, Northern Ireland and Eire (Audini *et al.* 2001).

Training for doctors in the psychiatry of old age was encouraged by the government when, in 1981, it authorised additional posts at senior registrar level, specifically to improve opportunities for such training (Secretary of State for Social Services, Secretary of State for Scotland, Secretary of State for Wales and Secretary of State for Northern Ireland 1981)

A further significant development in the recognition of mental health services for older people as a specialty was the creation of a specialist group by the Royal College of Psychiatrists. In 1973 Felix Post became the first chairman of a group for the psychiatry of old age in the college. In 1978 this acquired the full status of a specialist section, and this section formed the professional focus for the development of 'psychogeriatrics' in Britain (Arie 1989).

Liaison between old age psychiatrists and geriatricians

Throughout the period in question, stress has been placed on the importance of liaison between psychiatrists and geriatricians, and the result of a lack of such liaison. It was argued that problems in service provision arose not solely from shortage of beds, but also from the use to which the available beds were put, and that this could be improved by better liaison between geriatricians and psychiatrists (Kay *et al.* 1966).

The Hospital Advisory Service Annual Report for 1974 highlighted almost universal difficulties in arranging hospital admissions for acutely disturbed older patients. As well as a lack of suitable accommodation for the initial management of these patients, psychiatrists and geriatricians sometimes disagreed about their responsibilities, resulting in deadlock. Some districts overcame these difficulties by the consultants concerned agreeing their responsibilities for certain categories of patient. In cases of uncertainty, patients were admitted to either a joint psychiatric/geriatric ward under the management of the psychiatrist or geriatrician, or into a similar smaller unit in the department of geriatrics or psychiatry, where similar joint management took place (National Health Service 1975).

Improved collaboration between geriatric medicine and old age psychiatry were considered to be essential for good patient care, efficient use of resources and effective planning and liaison with other services. Such collaboration was encouraged by the Royal College of Physicians and the Royal College of Psychiatrists (1989), who also advocated consideration of more joint departments. Arie's department in Nottingham has been referred to as an example: here, physicians and psychiatrists were equal partners in what was described as an integrated joint enterprise. Although services were differentiated, there were cross-training initiatives and constant formal and informal collaboration and support (Arie 1990).

However, in visits to 10 services in England, Shulman and Arie (1991) found that effective working links between the two specialties existed in the minority of cases. While collaboration with geriatric medical services was a universally accepted principle, it was practised by surprisingly few services, even in general hospital settings. In the majority of services, cordial but somewhat distant relationships existed. Reciprocal individual consultations were the rule, rather than collaboration across the board. In only two of the 10 services (Nottingham, Crewe) could it be said that there was true collaboration.

Reasons put forward for this lack of close working include attitudinal and administrative distance between specialties, and the personalities of individuals (Jolley and Arie 1992). Health service organisation has also been suggested as a contributory factor. Where there was only one consultant old age psychiatrist to three or four consultant geriatricians, interaction between even these closely allied colleagues was superficial. The relationship started to change, however, as geriatric medicine consolidated rather than expanded its human resources, and ratios of 1:1 became possible.

A further contributing feature was the realignment of geriatric medicine with general medicine in many acute NHS trusts created in the 1990s. Driven by a desire to make new investigations and modern treatment available to all patients, irrespective of age, and to bring together the skills of both medical disciplines, this movement sometimes seemed to be at the expense of commitment to those patients with complex multiple pathology who required long-term rehabilitation and supportive efforts, in conjunction with colleagues (including old age psychiatry services). Many specialist geriatric services spent less time in community activities than they had done a decade previously, and this was not something with which specialist old age psychiatry felt comfortable (Arie and Jolley 1998).

Creation of specialist assessment units

An important factor in the development of mental health services for older people was the creation of specialist assessment units in hospitals. The case for such units included the benefits for the whole service of effective assessment of patients at an early stage, and avoidance of misplacement of patients (Arie and Isaacs 1978).

Robinson (1962) described an early version of such a unit, a 'geriatric admission unit' at Crichton Royal Hospital. The unit, opened in 1958, dealt with all health service admissions of patients aged 65 years and over, of which there were approximately 150 a year. There were two reception wards, each with 20 beds. Patients suffering from mainly depressive disorders spent an average of 8–10 weeks in the short-stay ward, while those with dementia or who were confused stayed 3–6 months in the medium-stay ward. If discharge was not in sight at the end of this period the patient was transferred to a long-stay ward, of which there were two, each with approximately 60 beds.

Assessment wards were considered the most effective way of achieving integration within the hospital service, which would in turn have favourable repercussions throughout the whole field of geriatric care. It was argued that these wards should be comprehensive, implying that the service should possess the equipment and staff needed to investigate all aspects of the older person's health and circumstances – physical, social and psychiatric. Important features were that the wards should be attached to the main district general or teaching hospital, staffed by both physicians and psychiatrists, supported by adjacent outpatient and day hospital facilities, and closely integrated, perhaps by joint appointments, with the local authority health and welfare departments, and with the general practitioner (GP) service (Kay *et al.* 1966).

Despite guidance in Hospital Memorandum HM(70)11: *Psycho-Geriatric Assessment Units* (Department of Health and Social Security 1970b) in which regional hospital boards were asked to provide a psychogeriatric assessment unit of 10 to 20 beds in each proposed district general hospital, by the late 1970s, joint assessment units had not yet been widely established, and they had sometimes become effectively the responsibility of either geriatric or psychiatric, rather than of both services (reference taken from Arie and Isaacs 1978).

Where such units did exist, it was considered important that they should offer treatment as well as assessment. A psychiatric 'admission ward' was perhaps a more appropriate concept than an assessment unit (Arie and Jolley 1982).

Practice has varied as to whether such an admission ward should accept the whole range of mental disorders in old age, perhaps placing patients with organic, and with functional mental illness, in sub-areas of the same ward, or whether these patients should be admitted to separate wards, with the option of older people with functional mental disorders of old age being nursed with younger psychiatrically ill patients. It has been argued that this must depend on the nature of local facilities, and that some segregation was desirable. Day space was also thought to be essential, making it easier to organise time and activities appropriate to groups with differing needs (Arie and Jolley 1982, 1998).

The multidisciplinary team

The importance of the multidisciplinary team has been promoted throughout the period in question, although, in line with the gradual emergence of the specialty, the role of some professions in relation to this client group has itself developed gradually. Professionals recognised as relevant to the team were old age psychiatrists, nurses, social workers, allied health professionals, such as physiotherapists, and clinical psychologists. Later additions to the list were community psychiatric nurses, occupational therapists, nurse and therapy managers, administrators, speech therapists, chiropodists and clinical pharmacists. Clearly, not all these professionals would be full-time members of the team (Department of Health and Social Security 1975; NHS Health Advisory Service 1982; Spencer and Jolley 1999). The *National Service Framework for Older People* (Department of Health 2001c), in line with the, by then, identified need for greater integration within primary care, and between health and other agencies, stated that specialist mental health services for older people should also have agreed working and referral arrangements with, amongst others, dietitians, district nurses, health visitors, trained bilingual or multilingual co-workers, and housing workers. Despite the acceptance of the model, there is still some way to go to ensure its application nationwide. In 2002, specialist multidisciplinary teams for older people with mental health problems existed in fewer than half of 70 areas audited, although they did partly exist in a further third (Audit Commission 2002).

The part played by clinical psychologists in mental health services for older people has been increasingly recognised. The appointment of the first psychologists with full-time posts for work with older people occurred in the 1970s. The Psychologists' Special Interest Group – Elderly (PSIGE) was formed in 1980, and later became a subsystem of the British Psychological Society Clinical Division. It is now a requirement that all psychologists gain experience of working with older people during clinical training, under the supervision of an appropriately qualified supervisor (British Psychological Society 1995; Britton and Woods 1996). The role of community psychiatric nurses had also grown in importance by the early 1990s, to the point that some services relied on their judgement on decisions to admit patients to hospital (Shulman and Arie 1991).

The concept of teamwork in mental health services for older people was seen as one where people worked together across professional boundaries, and that, except where there were legal or knowledge-based constraints, roles overlapped and members of the team derived their duties from the assessed needs of the patients, rather than merely from their professional labels or from the prescription of the team leader (Arie and Jolley 1998).

The term 'community mental health team' became widely used, perhaps in line with adult mental health services, where this phrase was common currency. The role of community mental health teams for older people included: being available, initiating and continuing interventions, liaison with other agencies, and making things work for individuals and groups. A large district may have had several community mental health teams for older people, each based within its own locality and interacting with other community teams, for example primary health-care or social services, as well as with each other, and with teams associated with day hospitals, long-stay or respite units, and assessment/treatment units.

With regard to referrals, most teams accommodated systems which allowed GPs direct access to some of their non-medical professionals. Some teams encouraged 'open access' to all the team's activities and some organised initial assessments by any one of a number of professionals, but most retained a mainstream of referrals from GPs or other doctors to the team. Regular reviews with the local social services team were routine in most services, and individual general practices bene-fited from a designated link-worker from within the team. Regular review of known patients in nursing homes and residential homes was considered to be at least as important as similar support and monitoring of patients still maintained at home (Spencer and Jolley 1999).

The role of general practitioners

As part of the more prominent role given to GPs in the government's legislation and guidance on community care at the end of the 1980s and 1990, they were expected, under their contract, to offer a visit to those aged 75 or over to see their home environment, find out whether carers and relatives were available and to assess social, physical and mental wellbeing. Under paragraph 13 of the terms of service, GPs were under an obligation to refer on patients where there were problems needing specialist services, for example the assistance of a geriatrician, and also to provide advice to enable patients to take advantage of local authority social services (Secretaries of State for Health, Wales, Northern Ireland and Scotland 1989).

There was potential for beneficial change within the frameworks of legislation. Both dementia and depression are common in the older population and both are expensive and distressing illnesses. There were therefore strong arguments for training and encouraging GPs to learn how to identify and manage these syndromes, and to maintain up-to-date registers of who was in difficulty (Jolley and Arie 1992). There was not, however, a flood of extra referrals to old age psychiatry as a result of this exercise and some doubted how useful it could be. GPs often know their older patients very well, although there are conflicting evaluations of how accurately they estimate mental wellbeing. Many older people with serious psychiatric disorders are not referred from primary to secondary resources and this may mean that they are denied the most effective treatments. The need has been identified for specialist services with better resources to achieve closer relationships with primary care teams (Arie and Jolley 1998).

Over 1000 GPs (a 55% response rate) responded to a survey which formed part of a study by the Audit Commission of mental health services for older people in 12 areas in England and Wales (Audit Commission 2000). Of these, only around one-half believed that it was important to look actively for early signs of dementia and to make an early diagnosis. Many of the others said they saw no point in looking for an incurable condition – even though carers could be helped by early advice. In contrast, almost nine out of ten believed it was important to look for early signs of depression and make a diagnosis. However, research shows that depression is often missed in general practice, and usually not treated appropriately. The GPs who believed that local mental health services for older people were good were also more likely to believe in the value of early diagnosis. In subsequent responses of 8051 GPs in 73 joint investment plan areas in England (*see* Chapter 2) fewer than two-thirds felt that an early diagnosis of dementia was important, and the majority were not using assessment scales. In most areas, fewer than half of GPs said they had received sufficient training to help them diagnose and manage dementia (Audit Commission 2002).

The *National Service Framework for Older People* (Department of Health 2001c) referred to the over-75s check, stating that the Department of Health would need to consider with the GP professional bodies the best way of assessing the health of older people proactively in primary care, in the light of the new single assessment process and the development of integrated service delivery through primary care trusts (PCTs), and in the context of discussions about how the GP contract should develop in future to incentivise the delivery of improved service quality, as well as quantity, in primary care. The subsequent new General Medical Services (GMS) contract did in fact require GPs under GMS to provide a consultation to patients aged 75 or over who requested it, if the patient had not had a consultation in the previous 12 months (Department of Health 2003a). The milestone in the *National Service Framework* relating to a protocol for GPs for treating patients with depression and dementia may be seen as an extremely positive development. If properly implemented and effectively monitored, it should lead to more consistent identification and treatment of older people with these conditions by GPs. PCTs should use their role to ensure that GPs, and other members of the primary healthcare team, have appropriate training, that the necessary links are made and maintained with secondary care services, and that audits include mental health services for older people (Audit Commission 2002; Department of Health 2001c).

The importance of domiciliary assessment

The key role of domiciliary assessment has been accepted since the early 1970s.
The Department of Health and Social Security Circular 4/70, *Psycho-Geriatric
Assessment Units* (Department of Health and Social Security 1970a), promoted
multi-agency assessment of older people at home, wherever possible without admission to hospital. Similarly, government guidance in 1975, *Better Services for the
Mentally Ill*, stated that, since the physical uprooting of an old person was in itself a
traumatic experience and may intensify existing anxieties or create new ones,
assessment of mentally disturbed older people should, wherever possible, take place
at home or in outpatient clinics (Department of Health and Social Security 1975).
The emphasis on the importance of home assessment for all patients referred from
the community continued in the late 1990s (Arie and Jolley 1998).

Reasons for the importance of domiciliary assessment, which should be carried
out by the psychiatrist together, when necessary, with other members of the team,
were:

- psychiatric problems in old people are almost always problems of function – and
  of function in their normal setting
- home visiting enables not only the function but the characteristics of that setting
  to be observed
- it is extremely difficult for GPs to communicate all the information necessary to
  the specialist service
- an on-the-spot visit enables one also to speak to neighbours, local shopkeepers,
  visiting friends
- the process of moving an old person, especially an old person who already has a
  degree of confusion, may exacerbate that confusion and, indeed, threaten life
- hospitalisation of an old person may pre-empt wiser and more appropriate
  solutions
- the initial visit may also establish what are the likely resources, material and
  human, that may assist in eventual resettlement (Arie and Jolley 1982).

Home assessment is also very useful in identifying carer stress, which affects significant numbers of carers of older people (Richardson and Orrell 2002).

The role of day hospitals

The contribution of day hospitals to the care of older people with mental health
problems was acknowledged by the early 1970s, when, in the context of the task
of replacing large mental hospitals, day hospital treatment was seen as having an
important part to play in services for people with dementia, especially those with
mild dementia, but also for some inpatients with severe dementia. The day hospital
was considered essentially different in function from the local authority day centre,
where activity would tend to be organised primarily to meet the need for social
care (Department of Health and Social Security 1972). Day hospital care was

recognised as a feasible alternative to permanent inpatient care for users with a carer at home, and as a means of providing relief for carers. An adequate and well-organised transport system was seen as essential (Jolley and Arie 1978).

This form of care was, by the early 1990s, considered fundamental for meeting the psychiatric care needs of older people, providing an important link between hospital and community, and was universally available. Some services, however, were aware that for some very frail older people, the stress of transport to the day hospital was too great, and in some instances disruptive. Innovations included a sitting service, a travelling day hospital, and a support care unit (Shulman and Arie 1991).

Categories of attenders at day hospitals included patients from the inpatient unit, for whom the day hospital provided interim support towards full independence, those coping fairly well in the community, for whom attendance, perhaps one day a week, gave vital security and links to services, those requiring a short period of observation, investigation or treatment, and many patients with dementia, who presented behavioural problems, that non-specialist day centres could not cope with, and whose families could continue to care for them at home, provided they spent some time at the day hospital (Arie and Jolley 1998).

In addition to their role as components of the specialist old age psychiatry service, a further function of day hospitals was seen as collaboration with, and support for, other forms of day care available to the population at risk, including geriatric day hospital care and day care provided by social services, or the voluntary sector.

The nature of the day hospital with regard to older people with dementia, and older people with functional mental illness, has been the subject of discussion. In relation to people suffering from dementia who had family caregivers, it was argued that they required to be dealt with in special psychogeriatric units, and that the distinction between day hospitals as clinical treatment units and day centres as communal facilities was less clear-cut than elsewhere in geriatric medicine. It may be that, in so far as long-term continuing care can be offered within the health service, the most appropriate solution is to place inpatient, respite and day-care facilities for people with dementia within the same small units, permitting rapid, easy transfer of patients from one mode to another as the patient's condition changes.

With regard to people with chronic or recurrent functional mental disorders who require long-term support, however, the case for segregation may be less strong. Such people, especially if they are socially isolated, can be helped by a day hospital setting to achieve a more stable adjustment and to continue to reside at home. Some newly discharged from psychiatric inpatient treatment may be enabled by this form of care to readjust to the outside world and to regain their independence. In other instances, a period of attendance can provide a break for the patient's family or an opportunity for medical observation. Often, however, older people with depressive or other functional mental disorders can be satisfactorily managed in general psychiatric day hospitals, where a mixture of different age groups can be mutually beneficial (Cooper 1997).

In a survey carried out in 2001, 207 old age psychiatric day hospitals responded from an identified total of 440 in England, Scotland, Wales, Northern Ireland and Eire. 11 864 users attended the day hospitals, with a mean of 33 users per day hospital. 6602 people with organic mental illness attended, with a mean of 34 per day hospital. 5262 people with functional mental illness attended, with a mean of 31 per day hospital; 157 day hospitals (76%) operated a mixed service, catering for users with organic and with functional mental illness (Audini *et al.* 2001).

Due to the lack of studies performed in the area of day hospitals, there has been little evidence to suggest that the availability of a day hospital to an old age psychiatrist actually reduced the number of patients whom he or she deemed it necessary to admit to inpatient care. It has been reported, however, that as many as 40% of psychogeriatric patients could be satisfactorily treated in a day hospital setting. Although day hospital attendance may not have prevented or delayed admission, the quality of the lives of both the patient and the carer during the time leading up to admission may have been beneficially affected (Howard 1994). Audits in 70 joint investment plan areas in England (*see* Chapter 2 for details of joint investment plans) found that there was at least one day hospital for older people with mental health problems in each area. However, these day hospitals provided comprehensive assessments and short-term treatment in fewer than half the areas (Audit Commission 2002).

A further benefit of day hospital provision for this client group was the maintenance of morale across the old age psychiatry service, since rotational movements of staff between different wards and community teams occurred, and members of several disciplines worked in the day hospital as well as other parts of the service (Howard 1994).

It has been argued that day hospitals for this client group are not the best way of achieving its goals, since a day hospital represents a large investment in capital, for a building which is used only a few hours a day, recurrent revenue costs, and absorbs many skilled staff. The question has been raised, of whether other providing agencies, for example local authorities, voluntary agencies and the private sector could provide the same services more economically. Commentators have also noted problems with transport, which, as noted above, is fundamental for the success of day care (Fasey 1994).

It is the view of this author that under-use of buildings could be addressed by better planning of the location of day hospitals, so that they are accessible for users, and of the overall use of the buildings in which they are located. Transport difficulties should be resolved through effective planning of transport, and location of facilities, to minimise both the need for transport, and the length of journey time. While local authorities and voluntary agencies have an important role to play in day care, they still require adequate funding in order to provide a service, so that shifting the emphasis of provision from the health sector to them could be seen simply as a transfer of funding responsibility. If, however, the option presented by Fasey (1994) was pursued, of redeployment of day hospital staff to domiciliary work and work in day centres in the community, this would offer scope for valuable inter-agency work, where the skills of the various staff concerned could be used to good effect.

Location of facilities

Due to the combined physical and mental health needs of many older people, and the advantages of ease of access, many commentators agreed that services should be based at the district general hospital. It was argued that inpatient assessment and treatment wards should be sited in the same district general hospital as acute psychiatric wards for other age groups, and with easy access to geriatric acute wards. Outpatient clinics should also be run from the same site, with easy access to, or side-by-side with, geriatric physicians. Although in urban areas, continuing care beds and day hospital places would be appropriately placed on a district general hospital campus, in more widespread communities it might be preferable to locate both in places where the population was clustered (Jolley and Arie 1992). By the early 1990s, seven out of ten services studied by Shulman and Arie (1991) had some or all of their admission facilities in district general hospitals.

Support for carers

Support for carers was recognised as important as early as 1960, when Macmillan (1960) discussed the importance of providing timely and appropriate support to carers, to prevent their complete rejection of the old person. Surveys in both this country and the USA in the 1960s showed that a surprisingly large number of old people remained in contact with their relatives. On the basis of one such study in the UK, it was estimated that if it had not been for the care and attention given to sick and infirm older people by their families the burden of the health and welfare services would have been three to five times as great as it was (Kay *et al.* 1966).

Arguments for support for carers continued in the 1970s. There was considered to be a strong case for increasing community support for those carrying the burden of a sick older relative, rather than increasing the number of hospital bed places for older people. It was recognised that families looking after very old relatives required help and advice from social workers and relief from stress, especially by the use of day centres. Day patients with dementia were found to be a vulnerable group, with the most important factor affecting the patient's viability in the community being family support. A strong case was put for focusing social work support, day centre care and other resources on those older patients with dementia cared for by their families. Older patients with dementia living alone were seen as presenting a very poor short-term prospect for survival (Brothwood 1971; Bergmann *et al.* 1978). By the 1990s, support groups were available for carers in some areas, and the information, advice and practical help that they may need to support them in caring for an older person were recognised. It was acknowledged that they may have physical and mental health needs of their own, and some were entitled to be assessed in their own right (Carers (Recognition and Services) Act 1995; Jolley and Arie 1992; Department of Health, 2001c).

CHAPTER 2

An integrated approach to services

Background

As far back as the 1960s, the argument was made for an integrated approach between health agencies and local authorities to improve services for older people with mental illness. The theme has remained constant, and since that time there have been a number of examples of service planning and working that demonstrated various types and levels of integration. A continuing message has been that, since the physical and mental health needs of older people were so closely linked, integration was the only logical way forward. The Nottingham mental health service, for example, was integrated with the general hospital geriatric service and the local authority welfare department (Macmillan 1960).

An important motivating factor for a co-ordinated approach has been the growing number of older people, and the capacity of services to manage demand. Linked to this was the belief that it was not only the number of beds available, but the planning and implementation of a balanced service that was required. In 1966, it was estimated that, with 4.5% of people aged 65 and over accommodated in institutions, an increase of just 1% of older people requiring institutional care would be problematic. Again, integrating all services into a comprehensive and balanced geriatric service was proposed as a solution, together with anticipating the needs of older people and developing community services (Kay *et al.* 1966).

A further rationale for integration was the avoidance of misplacement of patients in geriatric and psychiatric hospitals. Misplacement can cause adverse effects, relating to the survival of the individual, and the chances of discharge from hospital. This topic was addressed by the Department of Health and Social Security, in Circular 4/70, *Psycho-Geriatric Assessment Units* (Department of Health and Social Security 1970a), which promoted multi-agency assessment of older people at home, wherever possible without admission to hospital. It stressed the need to prevent misplacement of older people, which could delay recovery and impede rehabilitation. One service, established in Cornwall to address the issue of misplacement, comprised a psychogeriatric assessment unit and geriatric and psychogeriatric long-stay annexes, provided by the regional hospital board, and three special residential homes, provided by the local authority (Donovan *et al.* 1971).

The replacement of large mental hospitals by other types of institutional settings provided a further impetus for the promotion of an integrated approach. Guidance was given for hospital authorities and local authorities to consult together to plan services in their districts, in the Circular HM(72)71, *Services for Mental Illness Related to Old Age* (Department of Health and Social Security 1972). This proposed a variety of forms of help and support in the community, including those from the older person's family, day centres, domiciliary health and social services, and residential care, which would need to be integrated with the hospital services. It also specified the need for arrangements for co-operation between hospital and local authority services, and for criteria and procedures for reaching decisions on individual cases.

In the late 1980s and the 1990s, there was much emphasis on the importance of joint planning of services and joint working, between health and social care agencies, and between these organisations and the independent sector, which incorporated both private and voluntary bodies. The aims of this joint approach included a more effective use of resources, and the delivery of a 'seamless' service, for people requiring health or social care, including older people with mental health problems, regardless of which, or how many agencies were responsible for commissioning and providing that care. The government White Papers concerned, together with the linked legislation, had a profound effect on services for all care groups, including older people with mental health problems.

Caring for People

The White Paper *Caring for People* (Secretaries of State for Health, Social Security, Wales and Scotland 1989) introduced policy developments which were intended to substantially strengthen the underlying incentives for health and social services authorities to work closely together. Two major aspects of this were funding arrangements for residential care, and the introduction of the Care Programme Approach (CPA).

The new funding arrangements for residential care meant that discharged hospital patients would have to undergo an assessment of their care needs before the 'care' costs of residential accommodation could be met at public expense. Health agencies and local authorities would therefore need to work closely together to arrange care for older people who were inappropriately placed in hospital, and to develop domiciliary and residential care packages.

The CPA related to people of all ages with a mental illness who were being treated in the community. All district health authorities were required to have instituted this, in collaboration with social services authorities, by 1 April 1991. The main features were that the needs of each patient for both continuing healthcare and social care were assessed before discharge, that effective arrangements were made as to how in principle those needs were to be met, including the maintenance of appropriate registers, and that a named individual was appointed to ensure that they were met in practice. In the light of the experience of the implementation of the CPA, it was revised in 1999. The revision established CPA as not simply an aftercare arrangement, but as a framework for mental healthcare, which was as applicable to service users in residential settings as to those in the community (Department of Health 1999a). The single assessment process for older people, as set out in HSC 2002/001: LAC(2002)1, *Guidance on the Single Assessment Process for Older People* (Department of Health, 2002a), which formed part of the implementation of the *National Service Framework for Older People* (Department of Health 2001c) replaced the CPA when older people with mental health needs were assessed and services arranged.

Caring for People (Secretaries of State for Health, Social Security, Wales and Scotland 1989) also acknowledged the important role played by carers, and argued that help for them to maintain their contribution to care, in the form of advice and support, or services such as day, domiciliary and respite care, was a sound investment.

The New NHS: modern – dependable

The end of the 1990s saw a change of emphasis in policy guidance, in line with the change of government. The companion White Paper to *Caring for People*, entitled *Working for Patients* (Secretaries of State for Health, Wales, Northern Ireland and Scotland 1989), had created an internal market between health authorities as commissioners, and NHS trusts as providers, of services. The White Paper *The New NHS: modern – dependable* (Secretary of State for Health 1997) described how the government would replace the internal market with integrated care.

Health Improvement Programmes, which would be local strategies for improving health and healthcare, led by health authorities, would be jointly agreed by all those charged with planning or providing health and social care. National Service Frameworks (NSFs) would help ensure consistent access to services and quality of care across the country. Primary care groups (PCGs), comprising all GPs in an area, together with community nurses, would take over from health authorities varying levels of responsibility for commissioning services, while being accountable to them. At the highest levels, they would be freestanding bodies – primary care trusts (PCTs), still accountable to health authorities; they would also provide community services.

From Vision to Reality (Department of Health 2001b), subsequently announced that Health Improvement Programmes were to become Health Improvement and Modernisation Plans, which were to provide the process and vehicle for three-year strategic planning across the local system and combine the need to address national outcome targets and priorities within the *NHS Plan* (Secretary of State for Health 2000), the NSFs and other national initiatives.

In the same year, EL(97)62/CI(97)24, *Better Services for Vulnerable People* (Department of Health 1997), in response to perceived difficulties in the multidisciplinary assessment of older people with complex needs, required health authorities and local authorities to work together, in partnership with NHS trusts, to agree local Joint Investment Plans for continuing and community care services. The plans were to include improvements to the content and process of multidisciplinary assessment of older people in both hospital and community healthcare settings, and the development of health and social care services for older people which focused on optimising independence through timely recuperation and rehabilitation opportunities. They were to concentrate on those services and individual needs that were at the interface between health and social services. Implementation was expected to be in place by 1999/2000.

Differences in funding mechanisms for health authorities and local authorities have frequently been referred to by those agencies as a stumbling block to effective establishment of joint services. This issue was addressed specifically in *Partnership in Action* (Department of Health 1998b), in which the government proposed to amend legislation to allow more flexibility between health and social services in three areas: pooled budgets, lead commissioning and integrated provision.

With regard to pooled budgets, the legislation would allow an NHS body and a social services authority to delegate functions and finance to the pool and to those authorised to access the budget. This flexibility would allow health and social services to bring resources together, to commission and provide services, in a pooled budget that would be accessible to both partners in the joint arrangements.

Under the proposal for lead commissioning, one agency, either health or social services, would be able to take the lead in commissioning the range of services for a particular group on behalf of both. One agency would be able to delegate functions and transfer funding to the other to take responsibility for commissioning both health and social care. This would enable staff in the lead agency to manage a single budget for commissioning both health and social care, facilitating holistic approaches and better co-ordination of care.

In relation to integrated provision, it was proposed to introduce legislation allowing NHS trusts and PCTs to provide some social care services, and also allowing social services in-house providers to provide a range of community health services. It was expected that the integrated provision approach would lead to the establishment of more 'one stop shops' (joint premises where users can receive fast and convenient services and advice from a number of agencies) and also encourage greater innovation in the training and skilling of staff working across the boundary.

The government's proposals were embodied in the Health Act 1999, which placed a duty on NHS bodies and local authorities to secure and advance the health and welfare of people in England and Wales, and made it easier for NHS bodies and local authorities to make payments to each other in respect of health and social care functions. It also allowed the creation of funds made up of contributions from both NHS bodies and local authorities in respect of health and social care functions.

The *National Service Framework for Older People* (Department of Health 2001c) set standards for the care of older people in all settings across health and social services. It included a specific standard for mental health in older people, although other standards (rooting out age discrimination, person-centred care, and the promotion of health and active life in older age) were also likely to have a positive impact on the mental health of older people, and services for older people with mental health problems.

The mental health in older people standard was:

Older people who have mental health problems have access to integrated mental health services, provided by the NHS and councils to ensure effective diagnosis, treatment and support, for them and for their carers.

One feature of the NSF, assessment, was, if properly implemented, likely to lead to both better integration of health and social care services, and more detection at an early stage of mental health problems in older people. An integrated approach by health agencies and local authorities in assessing the needs of older people had been encouraged by the announcement in the *NHS Plan* (Secretary of State for Health 2000) of the introduction, by April 2002, of a single assessment process for health and social care, initially for those older people who were most vulnerable. The NSF provided more detailed guidance, specifying that when older people attended primary care, or sought help from social services or attended hospital, either as an elective admission or as an emergency, health and social care professionals were to be aware that they may have needs, beyond their immediate problem. Front-line professionals were to explore whether these further problems existed. Where the problems appeared to be complex enough for a fuller assessment, the assessment was to consist of a set of standardised domains of need, which included mental health. The mental health domain comprised cognition, including dementia, and mental health, including depression.

Assessment might identify the need for more specialist assessments, for example a specialist medical need, such as cognitive impairment. If admission to long-term care was a possibility, full multidisciplinary assessment was to take place, to identify opportunities for rehabilitation and to reduce inappropriate admissions.

The NSF included, as milestones, that, by April 2004:

- relevant local plans developed with local authority and independent sector partners, should have included the development of an integrated mental health service for older people, including mental health promotion
- PCTs will have ensured that every general practice is using a protocol agreed with local specialist services, health and social services, to diagnose, treat and care for patients with depression or dementia
- health and social care systems should have agreed protocols in place for the care and management of older people with mental health problems.

The Commission for Health Improvement, the Audit Commission and the Social Services Inspectorate (subsequently the Commission for Healthcare Audit and Inspection, known as the Healthcare Commission and the Commission for Social Care Inspection) were to have responsibility for reviewing progress on implementation. They were to measure progress against the NSF standards, so that good practice could be shared and action could be taken where necessary, to improve services (www.chi.nhs.uk).

The scope for successful integration

Some of the policy initiatives described above may be perceived as positive: for example, the scope offered by the *National Service Framework for Older People* for improvements in mental health services for older people. It is to be hoped that these relatively recent policy measures, aimed at integrated service planning and provision, will prove more successful and sustainable than previous attempts, since, despite the progress which has been achieved in gaining recognition for old age psychiatry as a specialty, and in the acceptance of important concepts such as the need for integration, services for older people with mental health problems are still patchy and inconsistent across the country, and often fail to link together into a coherent service network.

Commissioners have a key role in setting priorities and targets for services, yet in an Audit Commission survey in 2000, health commissioners in only four of the 12 areas visited had definite goals and plans for the future shape of mental health services for older people. In most of the other areas, the service was shaped by providers, who generally had clearer views than commissioners about what should be provided and how it should be organised. Consultant psychiatrists usually had the greatest influence on the way services developed, except in two sites (Audit Commission 2000). In subsequent audits in 70 joint investment plan areas in England, of health authorities, including their PCGs, local authorities and trusts providing mental health services for older people (including PCTs), the Audit Commission found that nearly a quarter of areas had no clear service goal and plans, and they were only partly in place in another third. Standard, jointly agreed procedures between health and social care for assessment and care management were routinely in place in just a third of areas, and partly in place in a further two-fifths (Audit Commission 2002).

Similarly, information gathered by the Social Services Inspectorate from inspections and monitoring during 2002–2003 (Department of Health 2003b), showed that, in most of the councils inspected, there were major gaps in services for older people with mental health problems, and that, where good services existed, they were isolated and disconnected. An important issue was the frequent lack of clear transitional agreements and of organisational coherence between mental health and older people's services. Establishing multidisciplinary and cross-agency services for older people with mental health problems continued to be a significant challenge.

The reported lack of strategic planning by some commissioners may be due to a number of factors. Until recently, in some areas older people with mental health problems may not have been clearly identified as a client group by commissioners, meaning that there would be no basis for a strategy for older people with mental health problems. This is likely to be changing now, with policy initiatives such as the NSF. They may previously have been included with older people generally, and while this may encourage a holistic approach, there is a danger that the physical needs of older people would take precedence, because they are easier to understand, and may appear to be more pressing. Where older people with mental health problems are identified as a specific client group, the necessary information may not be collected and analysed by commissioners, in order to provide an accurate population needs assessment for the client group, which would form an essential part of the strategy. Older people with mental health problems may be included in different parts of directorates in health organisations and local authorities. For example, within one geographical area, they may be included in 'mental health' by one agency, and in 'older people' by the other, thus making a joint approach difficult. Whether or not older people with mental health problems are identified as a specific client group, within mental health services, the needs of adults of working age have historically taken precedence over those of other ages, i.e. older people, and children and adolescents.

If providers have shaped services, there would be potential pitfalls. They may not have used population needs assessment to inform development and organisation of services, so it is likely that the type, level and location of services would have been decided on the basis of historical patterns, rather than actual need. They, too, may have given precedence within mental health services to adults of working age.

Consultant psychiatrists have played a leading role in establishing innovative services, for example the domus philosophy of residential care (Lindesay *et al*, 1991; Dean *et al*. 1993). However, there are potential concerns relating to their having a large influence on the development of services. There is a history of lack of integration between old age psychiatry and general geriatric services, and the extent of liaison between primary and secondary care is variable. While promoting the importance of the multidisciplinary team, psychiatrists have not always enjoyed the close working relations on the ground with social services staff experienced by, for example, their nursing and allied health professional colleagues. It is, therefore, unlikely that colleagues from these other services would be influential in the psychiatrists' thinking, so that their service model would be likely to lack the perspective of these types of integrated planning and working. Consultant psychiatrists may also have competing research interests to consider.

A further factor likely to affect the success of integration is the frequency of changes in the structure of the health service in recent years, which has made it difficult for those involved to implement all the improvements envisaged to timescale.

PART II

OLD AGE PSYCHIATRY AS A DISCIPLINE WORLDWIDE

CHAPTER 3

Development of the discipline

From its beginnings in the United Kingdom (UK) at around the middle of the 20th century, old age psychiatry as a discipline grew significantly internationally by the late 1980s. The British approach to old age psychiatry has attracted interest worldwide, and been adapted to the health services of many countries. British courses in the 1980s, for example, drew participants from many countries, both developed and developing, thus enabling discussion based on the experience of services designed for the needs of different cultures. By the early 1990s, a pattern was established of speakers and practitioners making visits internationally, in particular between Europe, Australasia and North America (Jolley and Arie 1992; Reifler and Cohen 1998).

A survey was conducted (Reifler and Cohen 1998) of members of the International Psychogeriatric Association (IPA) to determine the state of development of both the profession of geriatric psychiatry and services for mentally ill older people. Ratings of each were based on a scale of 1 to 4, with 1 representing little to no development, 4 being the highest, and 2 set as the desired minimum. A questionnaire was sent to the entire membership of the IPA, asking each member to choose the stage of development that best represented the current situation in that member's country. Table 3.1 shows the mean scores for those countries from which there were at least five replies, and which are covered in this book (European countries, the USA, Canada and Australia).

The countries that had a mean score of less than 2 (the desired minimum) for the development of geriatric psychiatry were Denmark, France, Italy, the Netherlands and Spain. Only Spain had a mean score of less than 2 for development of services for mentally ill older people. The UK was rated best, with mean scores above 3 for both categories; Spain had the poorest ratings, with mean scores of less than 2 for both categories.

Results of the survey also showed that the developed countries had established training programmes and a broad range of clinical services, although no countries were yet at stage 4 on either the development of the profession or development of services. Many nations had only a few self-selected individuals with an interest in late-life mental illness, and no specialised treatment programmes.

With the exception of services for mentally ill older people in Italy, the scores reproduced in Table 3.1 are broadly borne out by the other studies (*see* Chapters 1 and 3–15). For mentally ill older people in Italy, a score as high as 2.2 would not be indicated, although, as explained in Chapter 4, the availability, and consistency of information relating to European countries may have contributed to this apparent discrepancy.

Table 3.1: Mean score for development of geriatric psychiatry as a profession and development of services for mentally ill older people, from selected countries (European, USA, Canada and Australia) with at least five replies

| Country | Mean score | |
	Geriatric psychiatry	Services for mentally ill older people
UK	3.1	3.2
Europe:		
Denmark	1.8	2.5
Finland	2.8	2.8
France	1.7	2.1
Germany	2.2	2.6
Italy	1.3	2.2
Netherlands	1.8	3.5
Norway	2.0	2.8
Spain	1.3	1.7
Sweden	2.5	2.8
Switzerland	2.4	3.1
USA	2.8	2.7
Canada	2.5	2.8
Australia	2.2	2.7

Adapted from: Reifler BV and Cohen W (1998) Practice of geriatric psychiatry and mental health services for the elderly: results of an international survey. *International Psychogeriatrics*. **10** (4): 351–7. Reproduced with permission.

PART III

EUROPE

CHAPTER 4

Difficulties in transnational comparisons

The task of the researcher in European health and social care issues has been made difficult by the lack of consistent data, and of measurable indicators. There has been, in general, a great lack of epidemiological data relating to morbidity and mortality in older people due to mental disorders (World Health Organization Regional Office for Europe 1979).

The (then) Commission of the European Community launched, in 1989, a cross-national project for the 12 European Community countries at that time, with the aims of analysing the provision of services to support the older population of 65 years and over, and sketching future developments and bottlenecks.

A major flaw in this first cross-national comparative study was the lack of uniform and measurable indicators. The fact that there was no uniform and widely accepted set of demographic data on the European population presented a serious problem for the study. Although most data collected and published by international agencies pointed in the same direction, the available figures sometimes differed significantly. This meant that population projections for the future needed to be handled and interpreted with great caution (Nijkamp *et al.* 1991).

An additional difficulty facing researchers wishing to undertake cross-national comparative studies on care services for older people has been the lack of uniformity and standardisation among concepts used. Even measurable indicators have shown a great variety among different countries, and some types of care service may have different meanings in different countries (Nijkamp *et al.* 1991). With regard to services for people with dementia, even the word nursing home has had a different meaning in various countries. The term dementia itself has had limited usefulness. Some commentators have found that medical diagnosis has been rather a poor guide to the disability resulting from the illness. Dementia appeared to be a mainly professional medical concept, whereas social services seemed to interpret this in terms of dependency. There was a great deal of documentation on policy and planning of services for dependent older people, as well as comparisons and analyses of these by member states of the European Community, inspired by, and closely related to, the field of gerontology. Much of this information, however, was difficult to find, as it was usually published in policy documents, was not in the scientific literature, and was often in the national language (Bleeker 1994).

A further source of difficulty has been differences in institutional arrangements. In relation to the care of older people in the European Union, the institutional arrangements for service systems may differ substantially. They may be governed by either public or private initiatives (or a combination of these), and private care delivery systems may be of either a profit or a non-profit nature. In general, the institutional arrangements (for example, centralised or decentralised) are not necessarily mirrored in similar arrangements for financing schemes, so there is a great variety of financial and institutional models for care services for older people. This issue has also contributed to the need for caution in making international comparisons (Nijkamp *et al.* 1991).

CHAPTER 5

Transnational comparison studies

Introduction

In this European section of the book, transnational comparisons by Bleeker (1994), Nijkamp *et al.* (1991), and the World Health Organization Regional Office for Europe (1979) are referred to at a number of points. As background information, provided below is an account of the main relevant findings from the World Health Organization (WHO) study. This is followed by brief descriptions of the Bleeker and the Nijkamp *et al.* studies, some of the findings of which are incorporated in subsequent pages.

World Health Organization study (1979)

The WHO Regional Office for Europe invited a number of countries to take part in a study of mortality and morbidity in older people, their associations with mental disorders, and the provision and utilisation of psychogeriatric services in the various countries. Nine countries participated at the national level (Bulgaria, Czechoslovakia, Finland, Ireland, the Netherlands, Norway, Sweden, the United Kingdom (UK) (England and Wales) and Yugoslavia) and the eight study areas selected for more detailed survey were: Russe, Bulgaria; Charlottenburg, Berlin (West); Helsinki, Finland; Dublin Ireland; Friesland, Netherlands; Skarborg, Sweden; Buckinghamshire, England; and Belgrade, Yugoslavia (World Health Organization Regional Office for Europe 1979).

Day services

This part of the study related to organised ambulatory services for patients aged 65 years and over, and more specifically to types of services given to older people in day hospitals, day centres and clubs in the selected study areas. In those areas where both day hospitals and day centres were provided, there was found to be little significant difference between the service given by each kind of facility. In fact, no differences were reported from Dublin, while in Helsinki only the absence of facilities for hairdressing and shaving in the day centres, and in Buckinghamshire the absence of bathing in day centres, distinguished the centres from each other (World Health Organization Regional Office for Europe 1979).

Residential care

In relation to organised residential care for psychogeriatric patients aged 65 years and over, the selected study areas were asked to give information about their provision of differentiated (special wards or units reserved for older people in which it was possible to relate the staffing pattern to the numbers of patients) and undifferentiated (in which all age groups were treated together, so that it was impossible to relate the numbers, or variety, of staff to the numbers of elderly patients) residential care. The most striking conclusion to be drawn from the information was that in most of the selected areas the alternative for mentally ill older people who could not remain in family care, or look after themselves, was the psychiatric hospital or the old people's home.

In Friesland, which had the largest number of people aged 65 years and over and 70 years and over, and where the population as a whole was distributed mostly in villages, with some in single dwellings, services for older people were provided mostly in wards in geriatric hospitals and in old people's homes or hostels; relatively small numbers were in psychiatric care.

Helsinki and Belgrade, with similar numbers of older people, differed considerably from each other in their provisions for them; the numbers in psychiatric hospitals were very different (Helsinki, 591; Belgrade, 270) and in Helsinki there were three times as many places in old people's homes or hostels. The use of boarding-out in family care as a means of retaining old people in the community was reported only from Helsinki (World Health Organization Regional Office for Europe 1979).

Overall conclusions on services

A significant conclusion from the study was that, if the results of this study were to be taken as a guide, the number of places in nursing homes for people with mental illness would need to be doubled. Another was that, if the patient's needs and capabilities as found in the study were taken into account, the essential requirement of the psychogeriatric patient would appear to be nursing, no matter where it is carried out (World Health Organization Regional Office for Europe 1979).

Training and education

Nine of the 10 countries approached provided tuition in geriatric psychiatry and geriatrics for medical and nursing students, and recognised geriatric medicine and geriatric psychiatry as medical specialities. Geriatric psychiatry and geriatric medicine were taught in medical schools in Bulgaria, Finland, Ireland and the UK

(England and Wales), and geriatric medicine alone was taught in Yugoslavia. Postgraduate training for specialists was available in Bulgaria, Czechoslovakia, Finland, Ireland, the UK and Yugoslavia. Little was known about specialist training for psychogeriatric nursing. In Ireland and Yugoslavia a small number of hours were devoted to such teaching, while in the UK eight weeks' practical experience was gained by student mental nurses. It was recognised, however, that in some European countries there was no specialisation in psychiatric nursing.

The findings demonstrated that, in the nursing field especially, a very substantial increase was required in the attention paid to special education in the field of older people, and that provision of further medical education should be increased. They also showed that, since family physicians would undertake much of the medical work in relation to older people, they especially needed, and would benefit from, further or postgraduate education in geriatric medicine and geriatric psychiatry (World Health Organization Regional Office for Europe 1979).

Nijkamp *et al.* study (1991)

As described in Chapter 4, in early 1989 the (then) Commission of the European Community launched a cross-national project to analyse the provision of services to support older people in the (then) European Community, and to sketch future developments and bottlenecks in this field. The project covered the 12 countries of the European Community (Belgium, Denmark, West Germany, Spain, France, Greece, Ireland, Italy, Luxembourg, Netherlands, Portugal, UK). The study, of people of 65 years and over, looked at both 'young elderly' (younger than 85 years) and 'old elderly' (85 years and older). The research examined care planning for older people, and was concerned not only with healthcare, but also with social, human and cultural aspects of wellbeing.

Bleeker study (1994)

In order to study psychogeriatric developments in Europe, a questionnaire was sent, in 1990, to the 151 members of the International Psychogeriatric Association (IPA) that were listed as responsible for either an institute or a clinical or research facility. A second mailing of 25 questionnaires was directed at a supposed key figure in psychogeriatrics in every country of the European continent. A total of 102 responses were obtained.

CHAPTER 6

Mental health services for older people in individual European countries

Introduction

This section describes aspects of services in nine European countries. As discussed in Chapter 4, accounts relating to more than one European country are affected by the lack of consistent transnational information. A further issue is the available literature, which both determined the choice of countries included below, and varied in its coverage of those countries. The UK is not included here, as UK services are covered in Chapter 1.

Belgium

In the early 1990s there was a shortage of care services, which was especially apparent for older people with dementia or other neuro-psychiatric problems, mainly due to a lack of care-intensive and specialised places for these patients. As a result, older people with dementia were placed elsewhere: 25% of admissions were to long-stay wards, 17% to old age homes and 15% to psychiatric hospitals. Half the accredited psychogeriatric wards were in general hospitals, and half were in psychiatric hospitals (Nijkamp *et al.* 1991).

Denmark

Denmark has taken seriously its responsibilities towards the growing populations of older people, and of those with dementia. Dissatisfaction with the conditions in existing mental hospitals led to the creation of a lobby to provide 'special geronto-psychiatric hospitals' within communities. As a consequence, 1345 beds were made available in five such specialist hospitals for the city of Copenhagen (population 110 000 aged 65 years and over) built in the 1960s and 1970s. These hospital beds were supported by day hospitals and nursing home beds, which were set aside for older people with chronic psychoses. It seems that good-quality specialist accommodation was designed with a view to responding positively to the needs of confused older people. The element of segregation from the rest of the older population was seen as having benefits for people with dementia. Community psychiatry services subsequently began to accept older people (including those with dementia) within their caseloads, and to work with day hospital and 'gerontopsychiatric' hospitals to help patients to remain at home if at all possible (Jolley and Arie 1992).

In the early 1990s it was declared official policy in Denmark that all services, including those for the most dependent people, were to be delivered in the older person's own home. In accordance with the shift from residential to community services, all residential and semi-residential services, like nursing homes and sheltered housing, were replaced by one category, 'flats for the elderly'. These flats, which were either in new buildings or conversions of existing facilities, were designed for disabled people, and flexible services were attached to them (Bleeker 1994). Despite these specific policy initiatives relating to older people, including those with mental health problems, psychogeriatrics as a defined branch of psychiatry emerged only very slowly, if at all, in Denmark (Jolley and Arie 1992).

Finland

In Finland, in the mid-1990s, psychogeriatrics was a subspecialty of psychiatry, and there were about 20 active psychogeriatricians. Many mental hospitals had special wards for dementia patients, with training facilities for carers. Community services remained limited (Bleeker 1994).

France

Psychogeriatric care in the mid-1990s, as previously, depended heavily on long-term clinical facilities, which were isolated from the community and unevenly distributed, leading to shortages in many places. Community services were widely available, but were usually not comprehensive. Admitting patients to a residential facility may also have been cheaper for carers (Bleeker 1994).

Older people who were admitted to residential care were confronted with the problems of misallocation and multiple transfers to other services. As a result, the psychological abilities of these older people were likely to diminish. A study of Caisse nationale assurance vieillesse travailleurs salariés (CNAVTS), which deals with pensions, in 1984 revealed that of 100 000 older people in long-stay hospitals, infirmary and psychiatric hospitals, 28% were misallocated and should have been cared for instead by home care or other suitable services (Nijkamp *et al.* 1991).

However, France has also had some innovative models of long-term care. Cantou homes, which were first established in the 1970s, were administratively autonomous small residences (about 12–15 places) for older people with dementia. The intention was that the older person's family was integrated in the activities of the group, if possible. The homes were located in the community, and had a stable staff, which undertook a variety of functions. Maisons d'accueil pour personnes âgées dépendantes (MAPAD) were residences with between 40 and 80 places for older people with physical or psychological handicaps (Nijkamp *et al.* 1991; Bleeker 1994).

Italy

In Italy, in the mid-1990s, there were several active groups of psychogeriatricians, mainly at the universities. The country had a large national research programme in ageing and took part in transitional studies on dementia. Services for people with dementia formed part of the overall picture of assistance for older people which was slowly beginning to be formed in the country, and there was a shortage of all services. In 1978, legislation had led to the closure of all chronic psychiatric facilities, which were replaced by community mental healthcare. Interesting and important developments in community psychiatry were the result, especially in the north. However, residential services for the most disabled patients, including people with dementia, suffered in quantity and quality (Bleeker 1994).

Luxembourg

Luxembourg provides an example of a European country which has achieved some progress in the provision of services for older people with mental health problems through specific planning. The government's Ministries of Health and Family devised a national programme relating to older people, which was accepted in 1988 (Goetschalckx 1997). Instead of simply increasing the number of beds in nursing homes to meet demand, they decided to reconsider the whole situation. They judged that it would make more sense, and be more appropriate for the needs of this population, to develop structures of home care. The main aim was to give older people the necessary support so that they could stay at home, in their own familiar environment, as long as possible. This led to a series of objectives, included in the 'Programme pluriannuel en matière de médecine sociale (1990)' (a pluriannual programme in matters of social medicine, devised by the social round table and the Ministry of Health. The social round table is a conference of representatives of private organisations active in the field of social medicine). In order to demonstrate the progress achieved, included below are summaries of selected targets set with regard to older people with neuro-degenerative diseases, with, beneath each target, an example of progress.

Progress against targets

Summaries of selected targets set in 1990 to improve health and social gain for older people with neuro-degenerative conditions, and examples of progress reported in 1997 follow.

1 *Extension and co-ordination of services.* The country was divided into five regions, each controlled by a regional co-ordination centre for older people. These centres were to advise people on the institutions and services available locally.

Progress

Having determined the geographical location of the various private organisations, the whole territory was theoretically covered for home care services. These services were separated between 'home help' (i.e. washing and grooming, housekeeping tasks) and 'home care' (medical care, like administration of injections, medical treatments).

2 *Development of intermediary structures offering options between staying at home and residential care*: day hospitals, psychogeriatric day care centres, service flats, family placement, financial help for adapting the home, moderating tax measures, and so on.

Progress

There were three psychogeriatric day care centres, specifically targeted at people with neuro-degenerative diseases. The Ministry of Family had integrated retirement homes, in which most of the residents were independent, relatively well people, and about one-third were dependent and needing a lot of care, for instance people who were independent at entry, and who became dependent over time. These often had day care centres adjacent to them; some had psycho-therapeutic units, for the care of people with greater difficulties, for instance people with dementia. These units were, however, not specifically adapted to this group.

3 *Creation of additional rooms in nursing homes.*

Progress

The Ministry of Health had significantly increased the number of beds in nursing homes, from 410 in 1989, to 814 in 1997 (with an 'urgency' waiting list of 1184 people). Another 180 were expected to be available by the end of 1999.

4 *Creation of beds for respite care*, to give family caregivers an opportunity to take a break.

Progress

Most nursing homes had to keep a few beds vacant for respite care, although sometimes these beds were being used for a permanent placement. The beds were very difficult to manage, planning was complicated and it was difficult to meet demand. The beds were also being used for crisis situations.

5 *Creation of psychogeriatric wards in nursing homes.*

Progress

This had been done: eight of the ten nursing homes had one or even two psycho-geriatric wards. Two of the integrated retirement homes also had special units. These wards were closed units. A problem mentioned by a few family carers was that the wards grouped people with dementia at all possible stages, which was rather humiliating or frightening for people in early stages. On the other hand, it might not be considered advisable to move people from one unit to another as the disease progressed.

6 *Global planning for the staff required,* with a particular emphasis on complemen-tary socially trained staff, for example occupational therapists, psychologists, and educators.

Progress

Every nursing home had a social worker and an occupational therapist.

7 *Clarification of the status of independent doctors in nursing homes,* for example making them salaried employees.

Progress

Some nursing homes now had doctors as (part-time) salaried personnel. This had the great advantage that the residents knew the doctor and vice versa, and that medical follow-up was done on a regular basis.

Commentary on progress

In the 10 years up to 1997, much was done to improve the care of older people in Luxembourg, although the specific interests of people with neuro-degenerative diseases only appeared in the margins. The major specific service for older people with mental health problems was the opening of the three psychogeriatric day care centres. They were, however, only accessible to people in the central region and in the region of Esch; people in the rural areas of the country were not provided with this opportunity. There were not many psychologists involved in the field of geria-trics in general, and in the field of neuro-degenerative diseases in particular. Family caregivers received little attention, apart from the provision of respite care. The Alzheimer Association ran a support group for family caregivers, and kept regular contact with the family if a person with dementia was visiting one of their psycho-geriatric day care centres. They also ran an Alzheimer helpline, for assistance and information around the clock (Goetschalckx 1997).

The Netherlands

The Netherlands has a comprehensive network of psychogeriatric services, both residential and community based. By 1991 psychogeriatrics had become the largest sector of mental healthcare. In the mid-1990s, psychogeriatric nursing homes played a major role in long-stay care, also providing day care services and support to community-based care. There was a tendency to reinforce home care by substitution of residential capacity. Case management was an option, to obtain the shift from institution-centred towards patient care-centred services (Bleeker 1994). In the early 1990s, nursing homes for older people (verpleeghuizen) were homes for the rehabilitation or permanent long-stay care of elderly patients. A nursing home could be a psychogeriatric nursing home for older people with dementia (psychogeriatrische verpleeghuizen), a somatic nursing home (somatische verpleeghuizen), or both.

Mental health advisory services (RIAGG) were regional institutes for ambulatory mental healthcare. The main activities were care, prevention and service, and older people were cared for by psychiatrists, social workers, social psychiatric nurses and psychologists (Nijkamp *et al.* 1991).

Sweden

At the beginning of the 1990s, it was felt in Sweden that only a small percentage of people with dementia should be cared for in an institution, and that most should be cared for in their own homes. The Swedish government wished to reduce the number of beds in institutions by half before the year 2000. To do so, resources and patients needed to be transferred primarily to home care programmes.

In the previous 10 years, paralleling the development of basic research concerning mental disorders in older people, there had been extensive development and progress in the institutional care and basic care of mentally ill patients. Generally, older patients with mental disorders were cared for in either psychiatric or geriatric clinics. In different parts of Sweden, however, psychogeriatric clinics, with multidisciplinary staffing, had been established. Alternative forms of care were also being explored. All over Sweden, day care centres for people with dementia had been created. Small collectives and sheltered housing units were also being tried, which were staffed 24 hours a day. These housing units were located in different parts of cities or counties, often in ordinary apartment houses, where two or three apartments were connected to provide room for six to eight patients.

By the mid-1990s, geriatric healthcare was highly developed, with several research centres of international standing, especially those concentrating on dementia. A whole range of residential and community alternatives had been developed, and were well-established for long-term care. They had grown away from psychiatry and geriatrics, which had increasingly focused on the assessment, reactivation and treatment of patients with dementia disorders. It was felt that for long-term care, continuous organisation under the responsibility of one medical specialty would be advantageous (Bucht and Steen 1990; Bleeker 1994).

West Germany

Information relating to Germany, which is taken from Bleeker's study, does not relate to the situation in the former German Democratic Republic, as there were no IPA members in that country at the time of the study, just before the unification of the country. In the western part of the country, which was affluent, the medical discipline was a strong factor in society, mainly autonomous or associated with clinical facilities. In relation to psychogeriatrics, outpatient services were being developed in several places, and networks were being established of various disciplines involved in care and research. Services included residential facilities of the medical (psychiatry, geriatrics) type for the most disabled patients, and those that were multidisciplinary in character, as in nursing homes and 'multi-level homes for the elderly'. There was a strong wish for more community support services to circumvent the necessity of institutionalisation (Bleeker 1994). At the beginning of the 1990s, there were nursing homes for older people with dementia (Geronto-psychiatrisches Pflegeheim), which were institutions accepted by the government. They offered housing, meal and health services, psychiatric care and therapy (Nijkamp *et al.* 1991).

Main features of services in individual European countries

Table 6.1 summarises the main features of services for older people with mental health problems, as described in relation to the nine countries listed above.

Due to the constraints in transnational comparisons mentioned in Chapter 4, care needs to be taken in the interpretation of this information. Nevertheless, with some details from nine countries, an impression may be gained of similarities and differences between these countries. Four had psychogeriatric wards, located in general or psychiatric hospitals, nursing homes or elsewhere. Four had innovative forms of residential care: either flats with support attached, small residences with family involvement, retirement homes catering for both dependent and non-dependent people, or units in ordinary apartment houses.

Community psychiatric services and research were mentioned in connection with three countries. With regard to psychogeriatric hospitals or clinics, and psychogeriatric nursing homes, these were mentioned in connection with only two countries in each case.

In relation to respite beds and intermediary structures, these were mentioned in connection with only one country in each case. It should be noted, however, that 'intermediary structures' (Luxembourg: offering options between staying at home and residential care) included day services, which were available in some other countries.

Assuming that the number of types of service mentioned in the available literature gives an indication of the level of comprehensiveness of services for older people with mental health problems, Luxembourg had four types of service

Table 6.1: Selected features of services for older people with mental health problems in nine European countries, 1990–1997.

	Belgium	Denmark	Finland	France	Italy	Luxembourg	Netherlands	Sweden	W Germany
Psychogeriatric wards	✓		✓	✓		✓			
Psychogeriatric hospitals/clinics		✓						✓	
Innovative residential care		✓		✓		✓		✓	
Psychogeriatric nursing home							✓		✓
Community psychiatric services		✓		✓			✓		
Respite beds						✓			
Intermediary structures*						✓			
Research					✓			✓	✓

* Offering options between staying at home and residential care.

mentioned, and Denmark, France and Sweden each had three types. For The Netherlands and West Germany, two types of service were included. With regard to Belgium, Finland and Italy, only one type of service was listed. It is interesting to note that Luxembourg, which had planned specifically for older people with mental health problems, had the greatest number of types of service mentioned. As stated above, Goetschalckx (1997) described some problems with certain services, for example difficulties in the management of beds in nursing homes which were intended for respite care, and considered that interests of people with neuro-degenerative diseases only appeared on the margins. However, the progress reported by Goetschalckx in 1997 on targets set in 1990 appeared to demonstrate significant improvements in services.

PART IV

THE UNITED STATES OF AMERICA

CHAPTER 7

The legislative background

The federal role

In 1955 the Mental Health Study Act was passed, authorising an appropriation to the Joint Commission on Mental Illness and Health to study and make recommendations on mental health policy. The study report, *Action for Mental Health*, argued strongly for an increased programme of services and more funds for basic long-term mental health research. The Community Mental Health Centers Act of 1963 strove to achieve the goals of *Action for Mental Health* through deinstitutionalisation: discharge of most long-term inpatient residents as well as prevention of unnecessary new admissions. Deinstitutionalisation was predicated on the belief that community-based services would be readily available and that the need for institutional services would soon be minimal. The effect of deinstitutionalisation on elderly, chronically mentally ill people, however, was actually only a transinstitutional shift. By 1977, nursing homes had surpassed state mental health facilities in the number of patients with chronic mental illness. By the early 1990s, many inpatient services had shifted from state mental hospitals to psychiatric units in general hospitals, which were more appropriate to short-term, less chronic interventions.

Although the community mental health centers (CMHCs) created under the 1963 Act were initially organised as comprehensive care centres to provide services to individuals regardless of age, they gave little attention to older adults. After a trend towards providing services for special target populations emerged in the 1970s, Congress mandated in 1975 that newly funded CMHCs should provide specialised services to older adults, a requirement that was re-emphasised in 1978 amendments to the Act. Though CMHCs made some progress in expanding services to older people, neither the 1975 nor the 1978 amendments provided adequate incentives for full implementation. Thus, in the mid-1990s the proportion of older people served by CMHCs remained at 6% (Rosen *et al.* 1995).

In terms of services for assistance to older people in general, many were authorised under the provisions of the Older Americans Act, which was passed by Congress in 1965 and subsequently renewed several times. Most communities in the United States have a network of such services (Zarit and Zarit 1998).

When the Carter administration began in 1976, problems associated with inadequately funded programmes and the deinstitutionalisation process were clearly evident, especially the need to develop community services for the most chronically disabled patients. In 1977, Carter established the Presidential Commission on Mental Health, which found a need for financially, geographically and socially accessible community-based services that also served the needs of various social and racial groups. The Mental Health Systems Act of 1980, a product of the commission, provided for special staffing and co-ordination grants for CMHCs with identified ageing programmes. The Reagan administration took office one month after the signing of the 1980 Act and it was never implemented. This represented a retreat from earlier congressional commitment to provide community mental health services to older adults.

In 1981, the bulk of federal mental health services funding, as well as funds from many other health and social programmes, were returned to the states in block grants, but with cuts in funding levels. Other federal programmes on which mentally ill people depended were cut, including social services and housing subsidies. The block grant funding combined substance abuse and mental health money, while decreasing funding for both. Less money was available to provide needed community-based care. Channelling the funds through states increased state influence on mental health programmes, and federal, and thus national, leadership was diminished. The diminution of the federal leadership role was felt particularly in such areas as services, clinical training, and the sponsorship of national meetings and work groups to promote national policy leadership in mental health (Rosen *et al.* 1995).

The Nursing Home Reform Act of the Omnibus Budget Reconciliation Act of 1987

Omnibus bills, in which are packaged many, often unrelated, proposals, assumed a new importance after Congress adopted its Budget Process in 1974. Using that process, each year the Senate and House of Representatives adopt a budget resolution setting an overall plan for government spending and revenues. In many years, they have followed up with an omnibus measure revising government programmes to conform to the overall plan (Congressional Quarterly Inc. 1993). The Nursing Home Reform Act of the Omnibus Budget Reconciliation Act of 1987 dealt specifically with the psychiatric aspects of long-term care. One section of the Act mandated pre-admission screening of potential nursing home residents and screening of current residents, to ensure that patients with mental illness were not admitted solely as a result of their psychiatric disorder to long-term care facilities that received federal financing.

The Act recognised that older adults with psychiatric conditions were over-represented in nursing homes, and stipulated that nursing homes must screen patients for psychiatric illness. If a patient was diagnosed with a mental illness, then the nursing home was required to (a) provide appropriate psychiatric care or (b) deny admission to the individual and/or transfer him/her to a more appropriate facility. Commentators in the mid-1990s reported that, at the time of the passage of this law, 65% of older adults in nursing homes who had mental health problems did not receive treatment. For-profit homes tended to rely on bachelor's level counsellors, and government homes used psychiatrists, whereas non-profit homes used psychologists and social workers as well as psychiatrists. Although early estimates suggested that between 2.4% and 18% of residents would have been excluded from nursing home care by this Act, later reports suggested sharp increases in mental health service provision in nursing homes after the passage of this law. Nevertheless, there were concerns about service standards and about fraud.

On the whole, the issue of providing adequate treatment to the transinstitutionalised older mentally ill residents of nursing homes in the USA has remained unresolved. For these individuals, 'return to the community' has meant a shift from the mental health system to the long-term care system, reduced access to mental health treatment, a shift of care from the states to private sector institutions, and a shift of costs from states to a mix of federal–state (Medicaid) and private (patient and family) financing (Curlik *et al.* 1991; Knight *et al.* 1998).

The Elder-Care, Long Term Care Assistance Act of 1988, introduced by Representative Waxman (a Democrat, from California: D-CA) provided assistance for a full range of home care and adult day care services, and expanded benefits for nursing home care (Zisselman and Rovner 1994).

CHAPTER 8

Funding: Medicare and Medicaid

Background

The Social Security Act of 1935 was one of the most important federally legislated measures concerning older people. Included in the Act and its amendments were old age and survivor benefits programmes which provided some basic security for older Americans. Survivors' benefits were payable to eligible family members when a breadwinner died; those who could collect benefits included a widow or widower who was aged 60 or older, or a widow or widower who was aged 50 or older and disabled (Social Security Administration 1996).

Thirty years later, Medicare and Medicaid were established under the Social Security Act to provide health insurance for people aged 65 or older and selected others (Medicare), and for poor people (Medicaid). These programmes were based on an acute care medical model of providing relief from major medical costs. In 1995, Medicare covered 97% of older adults.

Medicare

Medicare has uniform national criteria and is not linked to income level. It is composed of two parts. Part A, known as Hospital Insurance, provides up to 60 days of full coverage for hospitalisation annually, certain extended care services, and home care. Payroll taxes deducted during the recipient's working years pay for Part A programmes, and there is no additional monthly premium. Part B, known as Supplemental Medical Insurance, has voluntary enrolment and carries a monthly premium that provides insurance for physicians' care and certain ambulatory care programmes. Under Part B, Medicare covers 80% of approved charges, and the recipient is responsible for an annual deductible amount, 20% of Medicare-approved charges, any additional amount that providers charge, and fees for non-covered services.

Medicare covers only 40–50% of the actual healthcare costs of the average older adult. Because Medicare was enacted with a focus on acute illness it, like private health insurance, lacks parity of physical health and mental health coverage. For example, the lifetime coverage limit on inpatient care in mental hospitals is 190 days; no similar limit exists for inpatient care in general hospitals beyond the standard maximum for any benefit period.

In 1984, the National Institute of Mental Health estimated that 51.2% of Medicare-funded mental health services went to disabled adults under 65 years of age. In 1988, 3% of the Medicare budget was spent on mental healthcare, versus 20–30% of private insurance spent on mental health. Medicare has spent very little on mental healthcare, half of what it does spend goes to younger adults, and the total outlay is disproportionately spent on inpatient care.

Changes brought about by the 1989 Omnibus Budget Reconciliation Act (OBRA) led to increases in Medicare spending on inpatient psychiatric care, including an expanding number of geropsychiatric inpatient units. Partial hospitalisation services for older adults exploded, increasing by 50% between 1986 and 1990. Outpatient mental health services increased by 20% in the same four-year period. Following the 1989 OBRA changes, one source of growth in outpatient mental healthcare was the proliferation of group programmes that scheduled and billed for outpatient visits to nursing homes. In combination, the increase in mental health services from 1992 to 1994 under Medicare was estimated at 25%, and Medicaid mental health expenditures showed a similar increase during the same period. This increase is, in part, a tribute to the flexibility of private services, which respond quickly to changes in the marketplace: in this case, the loosening of mental health payments at a time when both public and private insurance sources were placing increasing restrictions on medical services. Although mental health benefits were liberalised with 1987 and 1989 federal budget reconciliation bills, Medicare coverage excludes two important benefits: (a) custodial care for Alzheimer's patients and those not requiring skilled nursing care and (b) outpatient prescription (e.g. psychotropic) drugs.

Outpatient mental health coverage was improved in the early 1990s by the lifting of an annual cap, so that psychologists and social workers were considered eligible, independent providers; however, significant limitations remain. Unlike outpatient healthcare services, which are covered at 80% in Part B, mental health services are reimbursed at only 50% of approved costs. Mental health services in the home are generally precluded. Community services are not routinely covered by Medicare or by any other third-party payer. Although care for chronic problems such as dementia is not covered, patients with dementia who were hospitalised for other medical diagnoses can sometimes receive Medicare for home health services on discharge.

Fee-for-service Medicare reimbursement has the advantage of emphasising assessment and encouraging the development of services at several levels of care throughout the nation. The ability of fee-for-service Medicare to produce rapid changes in service delivery to older adults, by a wide spectrum of service entities with minimal administrative overheads is its greatest strength. On the negative side, Medicare regulations have tended to discourage home visits for mental health services, if not eliminate them altogether. Interdisciplinary co-operation in the form of communication with the primary care physician is encouraged, but such communication cannot be said to amount to working in an interdisciplinary team setting.

Medicare's emphasis on inpatient care tends to exacerbate the existing imbalance of older adults in inpatient versus outpatient care, and is bad mental health policy in any case, since outpatient care is generally more effective and less expensive. While assessment is encouraged, its accuracy may be compromised by the desire to increase income. In 1991, national data were used to show that the Medicare Diagnostic Related Groups (DRG) system had led to a doubling of diagnoses of major depressive disorder between 1980 and 1985. It was argued that these diagnoses were a result of 'gaming the system' – that is, the less serious, depressive spectrum diagnoses were changed to the more severe one, which justified hospital admission and longer treatment time. While the Medicare fee-for-service reimbursement model seems to have expanded mental health service delivery to older adults dramatically, it has encouraged the privatisation of mental healthcare for older adults, and encouraged inpatient over outpatient options.

With Medicare, the federal government has failed to take the lead in providing a model for mental health services to older people. Instead, the Medicare system has created financial barriers and disincentives for providers and patients alike, and discouraged mental illness prevention, early intervention and rehabilitation (Estes 1995; Knight and Kaskie 1995; Rosen *et al.* 1995; Zarit and Zarit 1998).

Medicaid

Medicaid, a joint federal–state programme for people with low income and limited assets, is the largest government payer for long-term care services. In 1995, Medicaid covered about 50% of nursing home services to older people, most of whom had some type of dementia or cognitive disorder. Means testing, which varies from state to state, is the basis for eligibility. Medicaid, combined with various demographic and other policy factors, was a key element in the shift from mental hospitals to nursing homes in the provision of services to older people with mental health problems. For older people with chronic mental illness or dementia, Medicaid offers primarily custodial nursing home care. Although outreach, prevention, early intervention and psychosocial services might prevent or eliminate the need for nursing home care among these people, and although nursing home care is a major financial burden for states, these services are limited, unavailable or even discouraged (Rosen *et al.* 1995).

People with low income who qualify for Medicaid may be able to receive some community-based services at minimal cost to them. The services that are covered vary from state to state. States may also have special programmes for lower-income people who fall above the minimum income levels for Medicaid eligibility. New Jersey, for example, provides assistance to families using adult day care for a relative suffering from dementia, while California helps families pay for respite care in cases of dementia, stroke, or other causes of brain damage (Zarit and Zarit 1998).

Other funding sources

Most communities in the USA have a network of ageing services designed to provide assistance to older people. Many services are authorised under the provisions of the Older Americans Act, which, as mentioned in Chapter 7, was passed by Congress in 1965, and was subsequently renewed several times. Services are also funded from a variety of other sources, including federal, state and local funds, and private donations. The result is a patchwork system of services which can vary from one locale to another, and which is not always co-ordinated within itself or with mental health services. The method of paying for services can also vary considerably: some programmes require partial or full payment by clients, while others are free or involve minimal costs (Zarit and Zarit 1998).

A principle of care for services to older adults is that they must be affordable. Until the early 1990s, most programme development in mental health services for older people took place in contexts that did not rely entirely on either fee-for-service or on Medicare funding, with the associated co-payment from the client. Other sources of funds included state funding for mental health services, community mental health system funding, training grants, research grants and various private, non-profit agencies. Programmes funded in this manner can provide service at little or no cost to the older client. These sources can be motivated by a perceived client need, interest in creative programme development, and training goals (Knight and Kaskie 1995). The Department of Veterans' Affairs operates programmes to benefit veterans and members of their families. The Department includes the Veterans' Benefits Administration, which conducts an integrated programme of veterans' benefits, and the Veterans Health Administration, which provides hospital, nursing home and domiciliary care, and outpatient medical and dental care to eligible veterans of military service in the armed forces (Office of the Federal Register National Archives and Records Administration 1999).

Managed care

Managed care programmes are systems that integrate the financing and delivery of health services in order to control medical costs and utilisation. Rapid growth in managed care, especially health maintenance organisations (HMOs), from 1980, affected the mental health system, including mental health services for Medicare- and Medicaid-eligible people. By the mid-1990s, approximately 10% of older Americans had opted to receive their Medicare-funded healthcare through HMOs. HMOs existed to provide overall healthcare management for a defined population. Since the HMO was paid per capita rather than per visit, it was motivated to achieve cost savings for its group of enrolees.

The implications of this growth in managed care for mental health and ageing has been a matter of considerable debate. There are no known successful models of HMO care of severely mentally ill older people, who probably need a different model of care. Some studies showed that managed care organisations had made respectable attempts to provide cost-effective, quality services for chronic illness. However, concern in the mid 1990s centred largely on two main areas: mental health 'carve-out' plans, and geriatric education and training. As a result of cost escalation for mental health and substance abuse services in HMOs, those insurers contracted with third-party mental health management vendors outside the normal benefits plan. These carved-out, contracted arrangements were shown to favour outpatient care, use less expensive, non-medical therapists, limit numbers of visits, and prefer less expensive group and family interventions. Not only were these methods of intervention not the most effective for providing mental health services to many older people, but they also lessened the opportunity for practising some of managed care's greatest assets: interdisciplinary team practice and continuity of care. The second major concern regarding managed care was that limits on specialised services and managed and closed systems of medical providers were disincentives to promoting academic medicine, research, and geriatric and mental health training to professional staff (Knight and Kaskie 1995; Rosen *et al.* 1995).

HMO enrolees had significantly fewer visits per user to specialty mental health providers. Mental health service users in HMOs were more likely to be treated by less expensive providers, and to receive the less expensive interventions mentioned above. In fact, the preference for group and family therapy in the delivery of mental health services was seen by some as a strength of the HMO model in application to older adults, as was the high potential for interdisciplinary, co-ordinated care within a single managed health system. However, the tendency toward carve-out, whatever the advantages for other populations and reasons, vitiated this advantage of HMOs for the elderly population.

Although there is no systematically collected evidence on assessment of mental disorders in older patients in HMOs, the complexity of accurate assessment in older adults runs counter to the HMOs' emphasis on use of non-specialised service providers. HMOs are weak in meeting the needs of mentally ill older people for specialised assessment, outreach and home visits. HMOs are not well suited organisationally for active outreach and case-finding approaches. When a guiding principle of an organisation is cost containment, seeking out patients who are not actively requesting services is counterproductive. In summary, because quality care for older adults depends on expertise in assessment and treatment, guidelines must be created to ensure that such expertise will be available. Without outside guidance, the managed care model is unlikely to engage in active case finding, provide specialty dementia care, or provide services to older adults with schizophrenia and other psychoses (Knight and Kaskie 1995).

CHAPTER 9

State policy and programme development

Background

The public sector has higher rates of service utilisation by older adults, and public agencies have been found to be twice as likely to provide outreach services as non-profit private agencies. However, with regard to programmes for seriously mentally ill people, while the public sector is capable of producing occasional examples of a model programme, these programmes rarely proliferate to the point of constituting a national programme of effective services.

While private sector services tend to be driven by money (in the case of mental health services for older people, the money is public money), public sector services are often determined by policies set by legislative committees, the executive branch and interest groups. With a few exceptions, activity in mental health and ageing at the state level has been driven primarily by the executive branch. The lack of a large and well-funded consumer or interest group lobby has been cited as a reason for the disarray of mental health policy for chronically mentally ill people in general, and for older people in particular (Knight and Kaskie 1995).

Federal–state relations

Since control of mental health programmes was shifted back to the states, they have increasingly left individual CMHCs with a reduced budget, and without any stipulation concerning how the money should be spent. In the mid 1990s, California continued the displacement of responsibility from federal to local governments by shifting control of mental health programmes from states to counties, where these services competed with the medical care system for the indigent as well as with police and fire services for funding.

The history of federal–state relationships regarding mental health in the USA has been characterised by shifting responsibility back and forth between the two, with neither level of government taking clear responsibility. With regard to health and social policies for older people, the federal system tends to lead to a wide variation in policy among states, and in some cases the absence of policy. In the mental health sector, this is perhaps most clearly the case with dementia care, which some states would include in mental health services, others would define as being in a different system, as its own system, or as not a state responsibility. The USA has a few model programmes for community-based outpatient services for older people, but lacks a system or a coherent national policy (Knight *et al.* 1998).

A barrier was created by congressional interest in returning to a block grant concept of service delivery, which lessened federal leadership in mental health and ageing. At the same time, most states have demonstrated no ability to develop national models, and their increasing reliance on managed care providers to deliver services has tended to exacerbate the fragmentation problem, and created gaps in public leadership in such areas as research and training. Block grant funding also exacerbated the problem of fragmentation of service delivery, and was counterproductive to the development of a continuum of care (Rosen *et al.* 1995).

Implications of legislation, policy and funding measures

The legislative, policy and funding measures implemented since the 1960s have had important implications for the nature and delivery of mental health services for older people in the USA. The main implications are described below.

Deinstitutionalisation of mentally ill people

One of the most significant changes in the mental health system in the past several decades was deinstitutionalisation, which began in the early 1960s when social security was expanded to cover the health needs of older people under Medicare and poor people under Medicaid. These programmes meant that poor older people, who previously resided in state mental hospitals because they were senile or similarly disabled, were now eligible for Medicaid and could be moved into nursing homes and board-and-care homes, where the federal government would share the cost. Both Medicaid and Supplemental Security Income (SSI) were to play an important role in enabling this deinstitutionalisation to occur. The SSI programme provided income support to persons aged 65 or older, blind or disabled adults, and blind or disabled children. Eligibility requirements and federal payment standards were nationally uniform. For people resident in institutions, the eligibility requirements and payment standards depended on the type of institution, although, with some exceptions, people resident in institutions were ineligible for SSI. For those in an institution for a complete calendar month, a fixed maximum federal payment applied where the institution received a substantial part of the cost of a person's care from the Medicaid programme. Other eligible persons in institutions could receive up to the full federal benefit rate (Social Security Administration 1999).

States began to shift older patients to nursing homes to promote cost savings in their programmes. The trend was significant: in 1963, among institutionalised older people, 48% of those aged over 65 with mental illness were in state institutions and the rest were in nursing homes. Six years later, only 25% were in state hospitals, and 75% were in nursing homes. In the general population, prior to dein-stitutionalisation, 77% of mental illness episodes were inpatient; the remainder were outpatient. By 1975, only 27% were inpatient, 70% were outpatient, and 3% were day treatment.

The exercise has been described as comprising both a process of transferring older patients to the community (deinstitutionalisation), and a process of transfer-ring them to other facilities such as nursing homes (transinstitutionalisation). Moreover, state and county psychiatric hospitals applied more stringent admission criteria, which reduced older adult admissions altogether. The discovery of more effective psychopharmacological interventions, and a desire to provide more humane care in the least restrictive setting, were claimed to be motivating factors in this movement, although, as outlined above, cost control played a significant part. Hospitals were full, and state legislatures were faced with the choice of building more or doing something else (Estes 1995; Knight *et al.* 1998).

Patterns of institutional care

In contrast to the often-stated priority of the mental health system for community-based treatment, in 1995 70% of all mental health expenditures were for inpatient care. This was a result of reimbursement policies of public and private insurers. After a deductible amount was reached for the limited number of older people who were eligible, both Medicare and private insurance reimbursed fully for hospitalisa-tion, again within limits. However, outpatient care was only partially covered, providing major incentives for the use of hospital care. In 1986, older people made up 8.7% of all inpatient, but only 3.1% of all outpatient, admissions. Commentators have described the predicament of older adults who needed mental healthcare in the 1990s as one marked by over-reliance on inpatient treatment, increased use of general hospitals as treatment sites, inadequate integration with the nursing home industry, and insufficient mental health referrals from general medical providers.

These patterns of institutional care resulted in part from mental health policy, and from what have been described as perverse economic incentives and multiple payers, that left the mental health system fragmented and unco-ordinated.

Older adults who sought care for mental health problems were likely to do so outside the mental health sector. It was reported in 1990 that only 56% of the service use for mental disorders by older people was provided through the mental health sector. These utilisation patterns may have serious consequences for older adults. The majority of older people who sought care from the general health sector saw internists or family practitioners, who as a group tend to overlook mental illness.

A further reason why much of the mental healthcare of older adults fell to family practitioners was that, because Medicare set the maximum allowable charge considerably lower than that for patients with other insurance, or those who paid out-of-pocket, many new and established mental health practitioners either limited the number of Medicare patients in their practices, or chose not to see geriatric patients at all. Primary care physicians, however, had the same economic dilemma as mental health specialists, and so themselves increasingly limited the numbers of Medicare patients seen, or reduced the average amount of time spent with such patients. Many primary care physicians relied excessively on medication, spent little time on counselling, and made few referrals to mental health professionals (Koenig *et al.* 1994; Estes 1995).

CHAPTER 10

Development of services

Geriatric psychiatry

In the mid-1970s, there was only one geriatric psychiatry fellowship programme in the United States; by the mid-1980s there were nine. In 1994, 37 such programmes applied for official accreditation in geriatric psychiatry, and at least 15 additional programmes existed that had not yet applied. In 1990, geriatric psychiatry achieved subspecialty status, and the first examination in geriatric psychiatry was offered, sponsored by the American Board of Psychiatry and Neurology. In 1995, there were approximately 35 000 psychiatrists in the USA, of whom more than 5000 listed geriatric or gerontologic psychiatry as one of their three primary interests in psychiatry. The American Association for Geriatric Psychiatry had more than 1400 psychiatrist members. However, only a few hundred had completed specialty training, and approximately 1000 psychiatrists had passed the examination granting them specialty status in geriatric psychiatry (Gatz and Finkel 1995). By 1998, over 2000 psychiatrists in the USA had passed the examination for certification in geriatric psychiatry by the American Board of Psychiatry and Neurology (Reifler and Cohen 1998).

Geriatric psychology

In the USA, specialisation in ageing within clinical psychology developed later and more slowly than in the UK. The first meeting on training psychologists to work with older people was held in 1981. A follow-up conference in 1992 provided mixed impressions of the growth of the specialty during the 1980s: university-based training showed little expansion although internship training, especially in the Veterans Affairs (VA) hospital system, had expanded.

The national organisation for clinical geropsychology in the USA was formed in 1992. Training for psychologists in ageing is not widespread in the USA (and not a requirement for all psychologists, as in the UK). The training models in the USA emphasise university teaching and research, VA or university medical centre employment, or independent practice as eventual employment opportunities in clinical psychology. Training and working within community-based mental health programmes has been relatively ignored, except for the use of community practice in training geropsychologists. Few psychologists with expertise in clinical geropsychology are found in community settings (Knight *et al.* 1998).

Only imperfect methods are available for estimating numbers of psychologists who serve older adults. For example, in 1995 there were 16 000 psychologists listed in the National Register of Health Service Providers in Psychology. A survey carried out just before that time of a national sample drawn from the register indicated that 10% of the average caseload consisted of individuals aged 65 and older. If specialising in clinical geropsychology was defined as devoting at least half one's practice to older adults and their families, then it was estimated that 4.4% of psychologists in the register, or just over 700 individuals, would qualify. Only a quarter of those serving older adults had specialised training in clinical geropsychology. The then recently-organised section for geropsychology in the Division of Clinical Psychology of the American Psychological Association had 238 members (Gatz and Finkel 1995).

The role of physicians

Physicians have been shown to be poor at detecting depression in medical inpatients, and outpatient service provision does not appear to have been any better. Studies have indicated that primary care clinician sensitivity to mental morbidity is low, and that primary care providers often neglect signs and symptoms of such morbidity in older people. Commentators reported in 1990 that primary care physicians tended to treat mental health problems only with psychotropic medications. These physicians were not likely to conduct clinical histories, involve family members with treatment, or to use psychosocial interventions. Another commentator claimed in 1996 that primary care doctors often misdiagnosed or overlooked depression among older adults. A survey reported in 1996 revealed that 26.4% of primary care physicians never evaluated the emotional status of individuals over the age of 75 (Zisselman and Rovner 1994; Knight *et al.* 1998).

Community mental health centres

As described in Chapter 7, the Community Mental Health Centers (CMHC) Act of 1963 financed the development of comprehensive community mental health centres. These centres were intended to provide services to deinstitutionalised mentally ill people, and to people who would have been institutionalised in the past. CMHC services targeted state hospital patients who did not require intensive supervision and CMHCs also served community residents who needed intermittent care. The centres provided comprehensive mental health services, including individual assessment, diagnosis and treatment in acute inpatient, day treatment or outpatient settings. Unlike the British approach, the American CMHCs were newly created agencies, rather than programmes reaching out from existing hospital services (Knight *et al.* 1998). The Community Mental Health Centers Act of 1975 mandated special services to, among others, older people, children and adolescents, and substance abusers.

With the passage of the Reagan administration's Omnibus Budget Reconciliation

Act (OBRA) of 1981, community mental health took a substantive turn. The initiation of a mental health block grant in alcohol, drug abuse and mental health (ADM) combined 10 categorical programmes previously funded on a project or state formula basis. This change transferred authority for the disbursement of federal CMHC funds to the states. Along with a reduction in mandated services (including the repeal of the mandate for specialised geriatric service), states were given broad discretion in the use of federal funds. Overall funding decreased by 21%, which reportedly led to reduced professional staffing, increased caseloads, service reorganisation to target chronically mentally ill and insured clients, and fewer services to children, older people and the uninsured, as well as to a decline in federal revenues being offset by state funds and private-pay clients. The impact of the ADM block grant was so significant that, after 1981, CMHCs were essentially redefined out of existence. According to *Mental Health, United States, 1992*, CMHCs were reclassified under the category 'ambulatory mental health organizations' (Estes 1995).

Community mental health programmes

Knight *et al.* (1998) reviewed a variety of mental health programmes for older adults with a range of mental health problems. The programmes included community mental health services in Spokane, Washington; Cedar Rapids, Iowa; and Ventura County, California; as well as a multi-service programme at Long Island Jewish Hospital in New York and a psychiatric consultation service to a federal housing programme for older people in Baltimore. The services spanned urban and rural areas, and used a variety of approaches to co-ordination of care. These programmes showed that it was possible to provide high-quality, community-based mental health services to mentally ill older people. The programmes also shared some common features. All emphasised accurate diagnosis of older adults, were interdisciplinary and treatment focused, and all used active case-finding methods and community education approaches to bring clients in. They also collaborated actively with other agencies that served older adults and, in three cases, with postal carriers, meter readers and other 'community gatekeepers'. All delivered mental health services to older adults at home. Mobile geriatric outreach teams, which used home-delivered services and interdisciplinary teams, proved effective in increasing service use by older adults in both urban and rural areas (Knight *et al.* 1998).

One way in which families can obtain respite is by hiring a home health aide or similar worker to come into the older person's home. The level of experience and competence of home health aides is quite variable, especially in relation to care of dementia patients. In some places, Alzheimer's Association chapters or other advocacy groups have organised respite care services to meet this need (Zarit and Zarit 1998).

Day care

In the 1980s, geriatric day care programmes existed, which were designed for people at risk who were mentally, physically or socially impaired, and who needed day services to maintain or improve their level of functioning so that they could remain in, or return to, their own homes. Such programmes also provided some respite for families. Cohen (1991) describes three models for such centres, categorised by Weissart *et al.* (1989).

- *Model 1* was situated in nursing homes and rehabilitation centres and provided services to physically dependent, older populations. Services included nursing, physical, occupational and speech therapies, and health and social services. Revenues came primarily from philanthropic and self-pay sources, with some Medicaid reimbursement.
- *Model 2* was situated in a general hospital or in a social service or housing agency. Most patients could perform activities of daily living, but more than 40% had mental disorders. Services included case management, professional counselling, transportation to and from centres, nutrition, education and health assessment. Revenues came mainly from governmental sources, particularly Medicaid.
- *Model 3* involved special-purpose centres to serve a single type of clientele such as blind people, mentally ill people or veterans. Daily costs were reimbursed by Medicaid, or were out-of-pocket.

From the mid-1980s to the mid-1990s, the number of adult day service programmes increased greatly. These were designed to provide structured activities and supervision for older people who had physical and/or mental disabilities, and relief to family caregivers. Programmes could vary widely in how they were organised and what populations they served. Some were organised on a medical model, were staffed by nurses, and had allied health services, such as physical therapy, available. In contrast to medical day care programmes, social models emphasised the benefits of social and recreational activities for their clients. Day hospitals offered many of the same services as inpatient hospitals, whereas adult day care provided less medical, psychiatric and rehabilitative care. Day care served a more chronically impaired population, and substantial functional improvement was not anticipated. Nevertheless, commentators in 1984 reported from a national survey of centres that there were benefits for patients (Mace and Rabins 1984).

Some day service programmes were designed only for people who were cognitively intact; others specialised in care of dementia patients. Most day programmes served both cognitively intact and impaired older people, and had varying amounts of special programming and activities for people with dementia. Some centres conducted almost all activities separately, while in other programmes, cognitively intact and impaired patients spent most of the day together, doing the same activities. These different ways of organising services for people with dementia cut across the medical–social model distinction. There is no consensus on which models of adult day services – medical or social, dementia-specific or integrated – work best (Zisselman and Rovner 1994; Zarit and Zarit 1998).

While day care could serve as a vital support to families in the period before nursing home care, a number of factors limited access to this resource. Lack of a stable funding source remained a pervasive problem. Transportation was another impediment to service utilisation. Elderly caregivers may be unable to drive, and clients with dementia may have difficulty entering buses or tolerating long bus rides. Not all individuals or families could benefit from day care. While the number of adult day care centres continued to grow, distribution was not uniform. Rural areas in particular were unlikely to possess a centre. Despite these pitfalls, adult day care programmes were an important component of the comprehensive services available to people with dementia (Zisselman and Rovner 1994).

Dementia clinics

Dementia clinics existed in the USA from the early 1980s, and provided a multidisciplinary assessment of the patient and the presenting family (Zisselman and Rovner 1994).

Voluntary organisations

One valuable source of information about local services for actual and potential service users, and for carers, is voluntary organisations, such as the Alzheimer's Association, or similar groups that focus on a specific problem or illness. In some parts of the country, there are unique arrangements for providing information and assistance. In California, for example, a state-wide network of Caregiver Resource Centers provides information and services to families of adults suffering from brain injuries and illnesses, including dementia and stroke (Zarit and Zarit 1998).

Inpatient care

The image of county asylums and state hospitals as custodial warehouses, where older patients are admitted and abandoned, appears to be out of date. Rather, most hospitals provide limited inpatient services to older adults, who are placed back to the community or another facility within a year of admission. In some places, the state or county hospital may be the only point of inpatient service. In considering policies surrounding community care, it is important to recognise that the county asylum and state hospital systems have changed dramatically. These hospitals have emerged as a form of community-based care, especially for older adults affected by psychoses, dementia and severe affective disorders.

From the late 1970s to the late 1990s in the USA, adult psychiatric inpatients moved from state and county facilities, to use predominantly general medical and private psychiatric inpatient hospitals. It was reported in 1993 that 43.3% of all adult inpatients were admitted to either a general hospital psychiatric unit or a scatter bed ('scatter bed' refers to individuals who are admitted to a hospital that does not have a special psychiatric unit or department), while 10.8% were admitted to a private psychiatric hospital. Knight et al. describe the work of Atay and colleagues on an examination of the Inventory of Mental Health Organizations survey which found that, after excluding those older adults who resided in nursing homes, 21.6% of all older inpatients were treated in general hospitals, and 10.6% were treated in psychiatric hospitals. The remainder were treated in state or county hospitals, Veterans Administration Hospitals, or by inpatient services affiliated with multi-service community mental health centres (Knight *et al.* 1998).

In terms of the kinds of treatment offered in state hospitals, it was reported in 1991 that 96% of the state hospitals had a floor, unit or wing designated for geriatric patients. Yet, just 60% of the state hospitals retained a professional staff member who was trained in geriatric psychiatry, and less than 20% of the hospitals provided any form of psychosocial treatment. These findings support the American Psychiatric Association's position that state and county hospitals rely on psychotropic medications and rarely use psychosocial interventions, even though well designed, multidisciplinary treatment principles have been formulated (Knight *et al.* 1998).

With regard to models for hospital-based care provided by the Department of Veterans Affairs (VA), in the mid-1990s VA mental health services, like the community-based programmes, emphasised accurate assessment, active treatment, and interdisciplinary services. Many VA mental health services were provided in medical settings (e.g. acute wards, chronic care, nursing homes) as well as in psychiatric units. Home care services were also a part of the VA continuum of care. Furthermore, VA played a major role in developing training in geriatric mental health across the constituent disciplines (Knight and Kaskie 1995).

Partial hospital programmes expanded significantly in the USA from the late 1980s to the late 1990s, and became a more common form of mental health service for older adults. These partial hospital programmes were organised under many different models, which offered a range of social and medical services (Knight *et al.* 1998).

Long-term care

Between 1955 and 1973, psychiatric first-admission rates for persons aged over 65 years declined by 70%. By 1980, persons aged over 65 years accounted for only 7% of psychiatric admissions; only one-third of these older people were aged over 75 years, and only 5% were aged over 85 years. The chief explanation for this striking change lay not in the introduction of new, more effective treatment methods, but in a mushroom-like growth and spread of geriatric and so-called 'rest' homes (Cooper 1997).

Between 1940 and 1980, nursing homes expanded tremendously in the USA, from 25 000 to 1 000 000 individual beds, as Medicare and Medicaid were initiated and included financial support for long-term care services. The nursing home population grew, as patients were supplied by the transinstitutionalisation of older adults from state psychiatric hospitals, a move which represented a cost-cutting strategy for state legislatures, who moved older people with mental illness from totally state-funded psychiatric hospitals to partly federally-funded nursing homes (Knight *et al.* 1998). In the 1960s, new federal regulations were instituted to construct modern nursing homes, and hospitals became increasingly more specialised in the treatment of acute illnesses (Zisselman and Rovner 1994).

In 1963, 48% of institutionalised mentally ill older people were in state psychiatric hospitals, with the remainder in nursing homes; in 1969, 75% were in nursing homes. The nursing home appeared to be where many of the former psychiatric hospital population would receive care: by the late 1990s, 50% of nursing home residents were demented, and 30% had psychoses (Knight *et al.* 1998).

Impact of the Omnibus Budget Reconciliation Act of 1987

Because of the large increase in the numbers of older people with chronic mental illness in nursing homes, the Omnibus Budget Reconciliation Act (OBRA) of 1987 established guidelines for applicants to nursing homes. As described in Chapter 7, OBRA 1987 required states to review the care of nursing home residents with mental disorders. If screening established that treatment was needed for mental illness but not physical disability, the person was to be excluded from nursing home care. In part because appropriate alternative care was usually unavailable, this screening programme did not meet its intended goal, and many nursing home patients were residents solely on account of psychological diagnoses or cognitive disability.

In fact, many older people in nursing homes still needed mental health services because of the strong comorbidity of physical and mental illness. OBRA legislation specified extensive requirements for addressing these comorbid mental health needs in nursing homes. However, research demonstrated that mental health needs of older nursing home residents were significantly neglected because of the disincentives that militated against providing such services. From the mid-1960s to the mid-1990s, medical care in nursing homes focused on chronic medical conditions, and not mental conditions, despite the fact that mental conditions had become among the most common diagnoses. Nursing home patients' need for psychiatric care had been uncertain, because of insufficient research on the prevalence of psychiatric disorders in this setting. Many nursing homes lacked psychosocial services, and overused physical restraints and psychotropic drugs in response to chronic mental illness, though the intent of OBRA legislation was to eliminate this ineffective, inhumane, custodial reaction (Zisselman and Rovner 1994; Rosen *et al.* 1995).

Alternative housing: foster care

For older people, particularly those with chronic mental illness, in need of care and protection in a substitute family, foster care could provide socialisation, stimulation, support and protection. The number of paying residents was usually limited to four. Evaluations of foster care programmes were favourable. One study in 1979 found that older people who were participants interacted to a moderate degree with family and community, and several investigators in the 1980s reported higher levels of wellbeing and equal improvements in activities of daily living functions versus nursing home patients. The cost of foster care was approximately three-fifths that of nursing homes (references taken from Cohen 1991).

Co-ordination of services

A starting point for identifying services for older people is the local Area Agency on Aging (AAA). AAAs were authorised by the Older Americans Act and are found in every part of the USA. In most states, the AAAs do not provide services directly, but serve as a clearing house, providing information about what type of help is available (Zarit and Zarit 1998).

An important step in providing support to frail older people in the community is co-ordinating mental health services with the help available from the ageing network. While there is widespread recognition of the need for co-ordination of services, the service system remains disorganised and confusing. There is no central entry point for services and little co-ordination among programmes. Often, the task of getting two programmes to co-operate with one another is monumental. They may have different eligibilities, assessments and reimbursement procedures. Clients find themselves dealing with multiple bureaucracies, each with rigid rules about service delivery. One worthwhile strategy is the development of links between community mental health programmes, AAAs and key providers of support services. These links lead to increased referrals of older adults to community mental health centres as well as access for mental health clients to appropriate community services (Zarit and Zarit 1998). Indiana successfully co-ordinated mental healthcare with an AAA. However, it was reported in 1987, from a survey of 281 community mental health centres across the country, that only 23% expressed a formal relationship with the local AAA (Knight and Kaskie 1995).

In the mid-1990s, it appeared that none of the health professionals and agencies involved in mental healthcare for older people had adequately addressed issues of collaboration, outreach, case identification or continuity of care. In 1995, in CMHCs, only 6% of clients were older people; among private mental health practitioners, fewer than 5% of clients were older people; and the professionals who provided most intervention for older people, acute care-oriented physicians, lacked training in both geriatrics and mental health (Rosen *et al.* 1995).

The many successful entrepreneurial programmes that had started in the USA by the 1990s may be perceived as positive. With no prescribed structure that had to be followed, anyone could start a programme. However, a concomitant weakness was the fact that no national, state or local body had overall responsibility or financial authority for service planning or delivery, and services were therefore unco-ordinated and uneven (Reifler 1997).

PART V

CANADA

CHAPTER 11

National guidelines for mental health services for older people

The recommendation to develop guidelines outlining the essential components of a comprehensive service for older people identified as clients, or potential clients, of mental health services emerged from the 1983 Colloquium on Mental Health Care of the Elderly, which was co-sponsored by the Mental Health Division, Health and Welfare Canada, and the Section on Geriatric Psychiatry of the Canadian Psychiatric Association. An outcome of the subsequent multidisciplinary working groups, which comprised members from different parts of Canada, was the publication *Guidelines for Comprehensive Services to Elderly Persons with Psychiatric Disorders* (Department of National Health and Welfare 1988). The characteristics of a comprehensive approach were outlined as follows.

Foundations of a comprehensive approach

1 Mental health problems and disorders are addressed in the context of general healthcare, taking into account the full range of biological, psychosocial and environmental factors which can affect mental health and functioning in late life.
2 Treatment and support services are mobilised in a co-ordinated manner from a wide variety of resources.
3 The level of care/service is closely geared to the level of need, as indicated by a thorough, systematic and ongoing assessment process.
4 A continuum of services, from minimal community support to full, specialised institutional care, is available. Patients should remain in the community as long as is feasible and beneficial.
5 There is sufficient flexibility to permit rapid identification of, and appropriate response to, changing needs.
6 The contributions of family caregivers, volunteers, professionals of many disciplines and other community resources are valued and supported.
7 The rights and best interests of clients are safeguarded.
8 The goal is to restore and preserve functioning, promote autonomy, prevent or minimise disability, and enhance the quality of life.

With regard to the necessary components of services, these were listed as follows.

Essential components of services

1 Consultation outreach team.
2 Outpatient psychogeriatric clinic.
3 Day programmes:
   • psychiatric day hospital programme
   • day care.
4 Psychogeriatric inpatient programmes for assessment and short-term treatment.
5 Rehabilitation and medium-stay beds.
6 Facilities for long-term care.
7 Community liaison education services.

CHAPTER 12

Development of services

In Canada, health services are planned, administered and delivered by the provincial and territorial governments. The federal government provides financial support through tax transfers. Through the Canada Health Act 1984, the government also ensures that all Canadian residents receive a publicly administered, comprehensive range of hospital and physician services, free of charge, anywhere in the country (personal communication, Allan Rock, Minister of Health 1999).

There have in the past been difficulties in establishing mental health services for older people in Canada. Based on the first year's experience of developing such a service in Toronto, Shulman (1981) considered that, from an organisational point of view, the lack of a catchment area for most general hospitals was an issue. Where no defined population was assigned to any one setting, this created major problems, and he and colleagues were attempting to establish independently a catchment area to identify the patients for whom their unit would be responsible. They hoped to demonstrate how much more efficient healthcare planning and evaluation could be when the area of responsibility was clearly defined.

There had at this stage been relatively little demand for the assessment or management of patients with dementia, and this was attributed to two factors. One was that the proportion of people aged over 65 in Canada was less than 10%, compared with over 14% in the UK, a demographic difference that was particularly apparent in those aged 80 and over. This population trend was expected to change dramatically within the following 20 years, when the number of those aged 80 and over in Canada was set to double. The second factor was that traditionally a poor service had been given to people with dementia by psychiatrists, most of whom had never viewed this population as within their sphere of responsibility or interest (Shulman 1981).

In a more recent example, in the province of Alberta, geriatric psychiatry was, in 1998, included by the provincial mental health board as one of four provincial programmes. The Alberta Mental Health Board (AMHB) replaced the Provincial Mental Health Advisory Board on 1 April 1999. The AMHB provided leadership in planning, delivered a continuum of integrated mental health services to Albertans, and acted as an advocate for mental health clients. In addition, the regional health authorities provided mental health services through psychiatric units in acute care hospitals.

The four provincial programmes were approved by the Minister of Health, to ensure that specialised mental health services, which were provincial in scope, were accessible and available to all Albertans, and that appropriate funding for these services was protected. Four Provincial Program Councils were established in May 1998 to develop the mission, vision and target populations of the individual programmes. In April 1999, the councils developed service delivery models for implementation, and in January 2000, the AMHB advertised for professionals with an interest in geriatric psychiatry to work in its services. The geriatric psychiatry programme targeted clients over the age of 65, whose most frequent diagnosis included mood disorders, psychotic disorders, anxiety disorders or dementia (*Healthbeat*, 1999; 2000).

PART VI

AUSTRALIA

CHAPTER 13

The policy background

Background

The decade from the mid-1980s to the mid-1990s saw major developments in policies for dementia care in Australia. The general policy climate in which these advances in dementia policy and programmes occurred was shaped by the Social Justice Strategy of the federal Labor government that held office from early 1983 to early 1996. Similar attention does not appear to have been given to other mental health problems experienced by older people.

Identifying the need for policy

Up until the early 1980s there was no co-ordinated policy. Responsibility for the care of people with dementia was divided up between various areas in a fragmented way, for example between the mental health system and aged care, between residential and community care, between formal and informal care, and between the Commonwealth and the states. Official Commonwealth reports on aged care written in this period did not even make mention of dementia as an issue (Commonwealth Department of Health and Family Services 1998, Howe 1997).

Prior to 1980, a major factor contributing to the assumption of greater responsibility by the Commonwealth was the scaling down of state government mental health institutions. States had progressively shifted costs to nursing homes as this alternative form of care expanded with federal funding made available from 1963. The federal government thus had *de facto* if not *de jure* responsibility, but there was little recognition of the needs of residents with dementia in the approach to care in most nursing homes.

In the early 1980s, the House of Representatives conducted an inquiry into home care and accommodation for older people, which was reported by the Parliament of the Commonwealth of Australia in 1982. The inquiry reported that care of confused older people was the single problem that was most repeatedly brought to the committee's attention. Many of the submissions were concerned with the problems that nursing homes had in caring for people with dementia, particularly those who were mobile or had behavioural problems. The inquiry concluded that action was needed to stimulate a diversity of provision in small units in existing nursing homes, and in a range of community psychogeriatric services, such as relative support groups, relief sitting and admissions, and daycare. Fundamental to all these developments was the provision of proper diagnostic and assessment services.

The Aged Care Reform Strategy

On coming into office in early 1983, the Labour government began to implement a number of measures based on the recommendations of the House of Representatives' report. The policies and programmes together came to be known as the Aged Care Reform Strategy, and from 1985, policy goals were translated into programmes at an unprecedented rate. The Strategy produced a number of changes in care of older people, including the expansion of community care, changes in the balance of residential care towards more hostel places and fewer nursing home places, and the setting up of aged care assessment teams as gatekeepers for residential care places (Commonwealth Department of Health and Family Services 1998; Howe 1997).

The Strategy gained added impetus from a Senate Select Committee inquiry into private nursing homes, which was reported by the Parliament of Australia in 1985. The need for more attention to be given to the care of residents with dementia was recognised in the recommendation that special programmes be set up within existing nursing homes for older people who were confused and mentally ill, including giving attention to the physical environment and staff training.

The Aged Care Reform Strategy presented opportunities for many initiatives that took their lead from the House of Representatives and Senate inquiries, while others built on innovations that had been pioneered by small groups of leading service providers and practitioners. The formal programme guidelines that were developed and the additional funding made available promoted these new ways of thinking about dementia care and their application in practice.

Home and Community Care Program

People with dementia and their carers were designated a special needs group under the Home and Community Care (HACC) Program, which commenced in 1984, and service providers responded in a variety of ways. Some opted to develop services specifically for this group, catering exclusively for people with dementia, broadly defined, but the more general response was for service providers to give more purposeful attention to the needs of clients with dementia and their carers within their general service, resulting in many different approaches. Staff training was one strategy that was adopted to improve dementia care across a wide range of services. In *Home and Community Care Program: Commonwealth priorities for service development*, which was published by the Department of Community Services in 1986, a statement of Commonwealth Priorities for Service Development noted that services had been encouraged to address access and equity issues for people with dementia (reference taken from Howe, 1997).

Hostel Dementia Grants Program

The major reform focused on dementia in the Aged Care Reform Strategy was the Hostel Dementia Grants Program, which encouraged the development of special programmes for hostel residents who suffered from dementia. These hostels in Australia were a form of sheltered accommodation that provided personal care and social support, but not the continuous nursing care that characterised nursing homes. Hostels offered a less restrictive environment for those who were mentally frail but still ambulant, and not needing a high level of nursing care (Howe 1997).

The Grants Program grew out of the Nursing Homes and Hostels Review, which reported in early 1986. Recognising the efforts that were being made to develop dementia programmes in hostels with limited funding, the review recommended that recurrent funding should be made available for dementia grants in hostels. The response to the Grants Program was very positive: in just four years, grants covered some 4000 places, and by 1991 it was estimated that half of the residents of hostels who could benefit from special dementia care were participating in the programmes.

Mid-term Review

The Aged Care Reform Strategy was designed to cover a period of ten years. In 1990 a Mid-term Review was carried out, to assess progress with the Strategy and develop directions for the future (Commonwealth Department of Health, Housing and Community Services 1991a and b). The Mid-term Review considered people with dementia as a special needs group, and recommended a number of specific changes to community and residential care programmes aimed at this group. However, probably the most significant recommendation for people with dementia was that measures be taken to develop an integrated national action plan, to advance dementia care within the overall framework of aged care policy.

The National Action Plan for Dementia Care

Putting the Pieces Together: a national action plan for dementia care, published by the Department of Health, Housing and Community Services in 1992, stated broad national goals for dementia care which were consistent with the goals of the aged care programme overall, and expressed the principles of access, equity and participation of the Social Justice Strategy that set the framework for all social policy in Australia. The Plan recognised that the aged care system was already doing a lot for people with dementia and their carers, and it therefore aimed to strengthen existing programmes and to identify gaps in service provision, where further action was needed. The approach taken in the Plan was to strengthen the capacity of existing programmes to provide dementia care and to support carers of people with dementia. It did not involve the establishment of a separate dementia care programme; rather, it weaved the strands of dementia care through the fabric of all aged care programmes.

The National Action Plan for Dementia Care (NAPDC) set national goals and targets for the period 1992–93 to 1996–97 in key areas that covered seven elements of the aged care programme. These are summarised below.

1 *Diagnosis and assessment:* Aimed at strengthening the capacity of health professionals who were involved in providing a diagnosis of dementia and assessing care needs of people with dementia and their carers.
2 *Services for people with dementia:* Aimed at developing the capacity of services to provide for this client group.
3 *Services for carers:* Aimed at supporting carers to maintain their caring role.
4 *Quality of service:* Aimed at improving education and training for those involved in providing care for people with dementia and their carers, and at producing materials designed to assist services to provide appropriate quality care.
5 *Research and evaluation:* Aimed at supporting the promotion, development and dissemination of research on dementia and dementia care.
6 *Community awareness:* Aimed at raising community awareness of dementia.
7 *Policy and planning:* Aimed at ensuring that policy makers included people with dementia in policy development and planning.

The Plan sought to improve the quality of services through demonstration projects, research consultancies and training initiatives. Activities carried out under the Plan included development of carer and staff training programmes, setting up of dementia counselling services, improved funding of research, and the funding of community awareness activities like National Alzheimer's Awareness Week.

An allocation of $31m was made for implementation of the Plan over five years. Two actions taken directly under the Plan were, firstly, the provision of extra funding in each year of the Plan to extend the role of the national network of aged care assessment teams in the diagnosis of dementia and assessment of care needs, and secondly, development of a resource and training package to equip assessment teams for this expanded role. A third initiative in assessment was taken as a consequence of the release of the report in 1993 of the Human Rights and Equal Opportunity Commission Inquiry into Mental Illness, which gave added impetus to advancing implementation of the Plan. In conjunction with the National Mental Health Program, funding of $12.4m over four years was made available in the 1994–95 budget for six pilot psychogeriatric care and support units. These units operated through aged care assessment teams, and supplemented state psychogeriatric services by providing support to residential care facilities in the assessment and management of residents with dementia and disturbed behaviour (Commonwealth Department of Health and Family Services 1998, Howe, 1997).

The Aged Care Act 1997 and reforms to the aged care system

The government introduced a package of reforms to the aged care system that were based around the unification of the former hostel and nursing home sectors. The reforms had their legislative underpinning in the Aged Care Act 1997, and its subordinate legislation, the Aged Care Principles, which came into effect on 1 October 1997 (Commonwealth Department of Health and Aged Care 2001). From that date, the funding and administration of hostels and nursing homes were restructured under one system, allowing aged care homes to offer the full continuum of care. The changes meant that residents could stay in one location if their care needs increased, provided the aged care home was able to ensure appropriate care. Services were no longer identified as hostels or nursing homes; instead, the legislation referred to residential aged care services. In 1998, the Aged Care Standards and Accreditation Agency commenced management of an accreditation process. Accreditation was linked to government funding, and aged care homes that were not accredited did not receive government subsidies. (Accreditation is discussed more fully in Chapter 18.)

CHAPTER 14

Development of services

The psychiatry of old age

It appears that the psychiatry of old age grew as a specialty in Australia from the mid-1980s. The New South Wales Institute of Psychiatry provided a 'Psychiatry of Old Age' course from 1985, included components on old age and disorders of old age in most of its many courses for health professionals, and held a number of seminars on relevant subject areas (for example on the 'confused and disturbed elderly' (CADE) units, which are described on p. 83. (New South Wales Ministerial Implementation Committee on Mental Health and Developmental Disability 1988).

In 1987, only a handful of psychiatrists in Australia had received advanced training in psychogeriatrics (Snowdon 1987). The Section of Psychiatry of Old Age of the Royal Australian and New Zealand College of Psychiatrists was founded in 1988, and by 1997 had expanded to embrace 10% of the college fellowship (Ames 1997).

Community-based care

In the mid-1980s, most older people with psychiatric problems were seen by general practitioners (GPs), few were referred to psychiatric services, and some saw geriatricians. Seeing GPs did not guarantee that psychiatric disorders would be recognised or, if recognised, appropriately treated (Snowdon 1987).

In Australia, historically, community care had received far less emphasis than residential care (Department of Community Services and Health 1990). A major departure from the past came when the Commonwealth government set up the Nursing Homes and Hostels Review. The review's report, which, as mentioned in Chapter 13, was published in 1986, was based on the philosophy that services for older people were provided in a framework of a continuum of care. Within this continuum, the emphasis should be on maintaining people in their own homes rather than in institutional or residential care, with services matched to care needs.

A major recommendation of the review was for resources to be redistributed away from residential care towards community services. Following the review's recommendations, the 1986–87 Commonwealth budget saw an expansion of the Home and Community Care (HACC) Program, mentioned in Chapter 13. By 1990, while community services received far greater emphasis than they had done in the past, funding of community care was still but a small fraction of that provided for residential care. Community-based care funded through the HACC programme was provided by local government agencies, voluntary groups and organised single service providers. However, the organisational network was extremely loose, and people suffering from dementia could easily fall through the net (Department of Community Services and Health 1990; Ames and Flynn 1994).

Day care

Day hospitals and day care traditionally included older people with a range of disabilities. However, in the 1980s there was a trend to develop day care programmes specifically to meet the needs of dementia sufferers (Department of Community Services and Health 1990).

Caregiver education

Because of the crucial role played by family caregivers in maintaining people with dementia in the community, there have been many efforts to help them through education and training programmes. Methods of educating caregivers have included self-help books, audio training courses and face-to-face training programmes.

   At Prince Henry Hospital in Sydney, Brodaty and Gresham developed a face-to-face training programme, which was arguably the most innovative of its type in the world. Their Dementia Carers' Programme aimed to reduce the stress on care-givers, to improve the quality of life of both dementia sufferers and caregivers, and to reduce the rate of placement of dementia sufferers in residential care. While the caregivers were being trained, the dementia sufferers participated in sessions of memory retraining, reminiscence therapy, reality orientation and general ward activities. Controlled evaluation of the Dementia Carers' Programme, reported by Brodaty and Gresham in 1989, showed that the full programme produced a reduction in the caregivers' stress levels not seen in other groups in the controlled evaluation. The programme reduced the demand for residential care: after two-and-a-half years, the dementia sufferers were only half as likely to be placed in residential care if their caregiver had participated in the full programme (Department of Community Services and Health 1990).

Respite care

Traditionally, respite care was based in a residential care facility such as a nursing home or hospital. By 1990, home-based respite care had been introduced, whereby the disabled person was looked after in his or her own home while the caregiver had a break (Department of Community Services and Health 1990).

Long-term care

The role of psychiatric hospitals

In New South Wales (NSW), during the 1960s and 1970s, plans were made to establish specialised units, including psychogeriatric units, in psychiatric hospitals. Progress appeared to be halted due to lack of funds and a reduction in real funding. In the late 1980s, psychogeriatric units still survived, some with close links to community psychogeriatric teams, although these latter served relatively small populations. As medical services became more complex and required more high technology, the medical aspects of the psychogeriatric service became more difficult to maintain.

In the late 1980s, because of a ruling by Justice Powell that dementia was not a 'mental illness' in the meaning of the Mental Health Act (NSW) 1958, and because of public fears and perceptions of psychiatric hospitals, more dementia sufferers than previously had been locked out of the services provided by the psychiatric system. Many were managed at home or in inappropriate nursing homes, often to their disadvantage and the disadvantage of their family and other carers (New South Wales Ministerial Implementation Committee on Mental Health and Developmental Disability 1988).

An increased role for nursing homes

In the late 1950s and early 1960s, a large number of nursing homes were established, and the Commonwealth government began to bear the increasing financial cost of care in these homes. Initially, selection criteria for nursing homes were very broad, and included many discharged psychiatric inpatients, and many people with dementia. This, among other things, shifted the onus of much institutional long-term care from psychiatric and geriatric hospitals into nursing homes. Patients who, for one reason or another, could not be managed in private nursing homes, or at home, continued to be admitted to psychiatric or geriatric nursing homes. The emphasis there was on providing care to people whom no one else would have (New South Wales Ministerial Implementation Committee on Mental Health and Developmental Disability 1988).

In the mid-1980s, about two-thirds of psychiatrically ill patients in nursing homes suffered from dementia, and at least one-third were depressed. Directors of nursing homes in the western suburbs of Melbourne estimated that about 10% of their patients should be in long-stay care because of their disturbed behaviour (Snowdon 1987). By the late 1980s, a relatively large proportion of people with dementia were in institutions. In contrast to the UK, where most people with dementia were not in institutions, in Australia perhaps half of those with moderate or severe dementia were (Snowdon 1987). From the late 1980s to the mid-1990s, older people with mental health problems requiring long-term care in Australia were far more likely to be in a nursing home or hostel than in a psychiatric unit or hospital. Nursing homes were designed to provide accommodation for people requiring 24-hour nursing care. By contrast, hostels did not provide nursing care, but were staffed to assist residents with particular tasks like bathing, dressing or eating. Hostel residents were, therefore, generally less impaired than nursing home residents, but there could be some overlap (Department of Community Services and Health 1990).

Falling bed numbers in psychiatric hospitals, and the parallel growth of nursing homes, had led to a situation where, by the early 1990s, no more than 5% of those with dementia were in long-stay psychiatric beds. Further factors likely to jeopardise the future of long-stay psychiatric beds were the decrepit physical state of many of the buildings, and a political climate which favoured deinstitutionalisation (Ames and Flynn 1994).

Dementia Grants Program

Although many special dementia hostels have been successfully set up in Australia, the more common approach has been to integrate dementia sufferers in standard hostels. As mentioned in Chapter 13, to encourage the development of special programmes for residents with dementia in hostels, the Commonwealth government offered dementia grants under which hostels could apply for special funding for this purpose. A study of the Dementia Grants Program in Victoria, reported in 1990, found that it was being used to help residents with dementia as intended (Department of Community Services and Health 1990). The Program had grown to provide over 6000 places by 1990 (Commonwealth Department of Health, Housing and Community Services 1991b).

Geriatric assessment teams

The Commonwealth gave responsibility for approving nursing home entry to regional geriatric assessment teams (GATs), with the aim of ensuring more appropriate use of nursing home beds. These multidisciplinary teams assessed people in their region applying for admission to residential care, and recommended nursing home or hostel placement, or additional community services, as considered appropriate (Department of Community Services and Health 1990). The GATs programme was introduced in 1984. The teams, each of which served a population of 10 000–15 000 people aged over 65, had a core of a geriatrician, community nurses, social workers and occupational therapists. By 1990, there were 106 teams, covering almost the whole country. The GATs' role was described as acting as gatekeepers to nursing homes and hostels, since they had ministerial delegation to sign the form that permitted funding for the individual to flow through to the institution, once they were admitted (Ames and Flynn 1994).

However, not all aspects of implementation ran smoothly. In New South Wales (NSW), by the mid to late-1980s, GATs worked in varying degrees of integration with geriatric services, and covered 50% of NSW. Because the state government was seen as responsible for psychiatric services, problems in relation to nursing home admission frequently arose, and considerable frustration and inefficiency resulted, affecting patients, carers and various health professionals. For instance, the relevant approval may have been disallowed because of potential aggressive or antisocial behaviour, even when the patient had been fully assessed by an experienced team and a nursing home director of nursing had accepted the patient. The patient may then have languished in an acute, expensive general hospital bed for long periods of time (New South Wales Ministerial Implementation Committee on Mental Health and Developmental Disability 1988).

The Mid-term Review and long-term care

The 1990 Mid-term Review identified three main issues relating to the next phase of residential care development. These were:

- growing evidence that HACC could support more dependent individuals in the community than was previously the case, reducing the need for hostel care
- supply side factors had inhibited the realisation of the planned upswing in hostel growth
- a wider range of retirement housing, including hostel-equivalent serviced apartments, had become available in the housing market.

Taken together, these factors suggested that the rapid expansion of hostels, as proposed in the Nursing Homes and Hostels Review, may no longer have been the most appropriate means of providing care to those whose dependency did not require nursing home care. It was felt that consideration should be given to adjusting the hostel ratio and making provision for more community care.

The projected increases in the prevalence of dementia in the immediate future was also a major challenge for aged care services. Action was needed to further the equitable provision of resources for dementia care in hostels, and more generally, concerted and ongoing policy development was required to ensure that provision of dementia care was advanced as an integral part of the aged care system. The review recommended that the provision of dementia care in hostels be extended to cover all residents assessed as needing such programmes, and that resources available for this purpose be equitably distributed (Commonwealth Department of Health, Housing and Community Services 1991a).

The 1997 reforms

As mentioned in Chapter 13, under the Aged Care Act 1997, from 1 October 1997, the funding and administration of hostels and nursing homes were restructured under one system, allowing aged care homes to offer the full continuum of care (Commonwealth Department of Health and Aged Care 2001).

Innovative models of long-term care

CADE units

The move towards deinstitutionalisation of psychiatric hospital patients created a need for alternative accommodation for the residents of these hospitals who suffered from dementia. In NSW, one solution was the setting up of a series of units for the confused and disturbed elderly (CADE units). The units were developed to meet the needs of a group of older people with behaviour disturbance of sufficient severity that they could not be managed in nursing homes, hostels or existing specialised facilities. They were designed to accommodate small groups of people with dementia in a home-like atmosphere. The first unit was opened in 1987, and was designed to accommodate 16 residents, with a staffing level equivalent to that used for similar patients in a psychiatric hospital. This staffing level facilitated the management of patients with significant behaviour disturbances. It also allowed the unit to develop a community support role for carers of people with dementia, and a consultative and educational role for professional and non-professional carers. The residents were found to improve in behaviour once transferred from the psychiatric hospital to the CADE unit, indicating that the new environment was more appropriate for them (New South Wales Ministerial Implementation Committee on Mental Health and Developmental Disability 1988; Department of Community Services and Health 1990).

Lodge programme

Among the pioneers of special hostel care for dementia sufferers was the Uniting Church in Victoria, which had a Lodge programme. The Lodges were set up in houses in the community, so that people with dementia could live as a family group under the direction of a supervisor. The need to maintain a harmonious family atmosphere meant, however, that dementia sufferers with problem behaviour could not be accommodated in this type of programme. Furthermore, while the principle of small group living was excellent, cost pressures meant that special hostels generally needed to accommodate a larger number of residents (Department of Community Services and Health 1990).

CHAPTER 15

Co-ordination of services

Difficulties in integration

Mental health services for older people in Australia have experienced difficulties in relation to integration of services. In NSW, in the mid to late-1980s, for example, the Commonwealth government provided funding through the Home and Community Care Program (*see* Chapter 13) for various services, such as community nurses and day centre staff. Much of this impinged on 'geriatric psychiatry', but there were problems, particularly in integration of geriatric and geriatric psychiatry services funded under the Program.

Overall, the provision of geriatric psychiatry services in NSW, though present and developing, was considered to be patchy, often poorly integrated with geriatric and other services, under-resourced, and precariously dependent on a few individuals. Definitions were thought to contribute to the problems. The definition of a patient with dementia as 'geriatric' or 'psychiatric' was often quite arbitrary, and the definition of the degree of behavioural disturbance was necessarily arbitrary. These factors contributed to confusion in the workplace, poor integration of services, multiple or no funding, lack of administrative cohesion, and increased stress and distress for the patient and the carer, whether family or professional. The problem was not between the geriatrician and geriatric psychiatrist in the field, but further upstream administratively. Lack of resources, and insufficient collaboration between disciplines and parts of the service, were important factors (New South Wales Ministerial Implementation Committee on Mental Health and Developmental Disability 1988).

With regard to the roles of the various professionals concerned, in the mid-1980s, few nursing homes in Australia were visited by psychiatrists, or received help from mental health teams. Few of the psychiatric wards for older people were closely linked with community teams who were able to assess, manage or follow up older mentally disturbed people in hostels, nursing homes or elsewhere in the community. In some places, geriatricians were primarily responsible for management of dementia without wanting to be – they had no psychiatrist available, and some patients were admitted to geriatric hospitals because no beds were obtainable in psychogeriatric units (Snowdon 1987).

Unlike Britain, where people with dementia who were mobile requiring assessment or care tended to fall automatically in the province of the psychogeriatrician, in Australia in the mid 1990s, uncomplicated cases of dementia were often assessed by the GATs. The psychogeriatric service focused its limited resources on dementia sufferers with behavioural disturbance, in addition to managing the functionally ill (Ames and Flynn 1994).

National government/state relations

In the mid to late-1980s, ambiguity of responsibility between the Commonwealth and the state was seen as a major problem in the provision of services. The state governments took responsibility for psychiatric patients at the turn of the 19th and 20th centuries, whereas the Commonwealth government traditionally took responsibility for geriatric care. There was therefore potential for discord and confusion (New South Wales Ministerial Implementation Committee on Mental Health and Developmental Disability 1988).

A decade later, a more positive image of national–state government relations emerged, whereby policies developed by states were complementary to national government plans. Some states had followed the Commonwealth in developing policies on dementia care. In NSW, for example, the state action plan on dementia, developed to cover the period 1996–2000, was complementary to the Commonwealth plan. The plan set goals covering diagnosis, assessment and provision of information, access to services, protection of rights of people with dementia, community awareness, and education and training.

In Victoria, a Ministerial Task Force on Dementia Services, set up in 1995, produced a number of reports which complemented the National Action Plan. The aims of these reports were to outline existing services and difficulties for people with dementia and their carers across the illness, make recommendations for changes to the service delivery system, provide sets of performance indicators for best practice for people with dementia and their carers, and identify training and service needs for service providers across the system (Commonwealth Department of Health and Family Services 1998).

PART VII

APPROACHES TO EVALUATING HEALTH AND SOCIAL CARE

CHAPTER 16

Background

Donabedian (1980, 1982) considered that an assessment of quality was a judgement concerning the process of care, based on the extent to which that care contributed to valued outcomes. These two features of care formed part of a triad: 'structure' referred to the resources used in the provision of care, and to the more stable arrangements under which care was produced; 'process' referred to the activities that constituted care; and the 'outcomes' were the consequences to health (Donabedian 1982).

In his view (Donabedian 1980, 1982), the process of healthcare was, itself, divisible into two major components: technical care and the management of the interpersonal relationship between the practitioner and the client. The interpersonal process was the necessary vehicle for the application of technical care, but it was also important in its own right, since it may, itself, be either therapeutic or hurtful, and because those who took part were expected to respect individual sensibilities, as well as the more general ethical and social rules that govern the relationships among people. The amenities of care were also relevant to the assessment of quality, though one had an option of regarding them either as properties of the care itself, or of the circumstances under which care was provided (Donabedian 1982).

Donabedian asserted that the outcomes of care that were relevant to an assessment of its quality should include patient knowledge, attitudes and behaviours, to the extent that they resulted from prior care and contributed to current or future health. Patient satisfaction was one such outcome. But patient satisfaction was significant also because it was a judgement on those aspects of the quality of care concerning which the client was the most trustworthy arbiter (Donabedian 1982).

Higginson (1994) quoted a number of commentators, including Donabedian, in defining evaluation of health services. Evaluation was described as the systematic and scientific method of determining whether a therapy or preventive act was successful in achieving predetermined objectives. Here, the formulation originally proposed by Donabedian was expanded, to comprise also 'outputs', and examples of the features that may be examined within each of the four aspects of care were included. Thus, when evaluating health services these could usually be considered in terms of:

- *structure or inputs*: resources in terms of human resources, equipment and money
- *process*: how the resources are used (such as domiciliary visits, beds, clinics)
- *output*: productivity or throughput (such as rates of clinic attendance or discharge, throughput)
- *outcome*: achievement of intended change in health status or quality of life.

Structural aspects influenced the process of care, so that its quality could be either diminished or enhanced. Similarly, changes in the process of care, including variations in its quality, influenced the output, and in turn the effect of care on health status and outcomes. Thus there was a functional relationship between these in that:

structure → process → output → outcome.

Organisational evaluations (the type of evaluation focused upon in this book) tended to assess the structure and process of care, whereas clinical and medical evaluations often measured the process and outcome of care. Standards of structure or process were most useful when these were proven to improve care, or if there was a very strong consensus that these were desirable.

The advantage of using generic measures of quality was that this allowed comparison of very different types of care. However, if the measure were not sensitive or appropriate to the aims of the care, for example for older people, then such an approach would not be possible. Even generic process measures may not be appropriate. Some of the generic nursing quality measures, for instance, had been criticised for poor reliability and validity, unwieldiness and obscurity in some of the terms.

The approaches to evaluation described in this book are organisational in nature; they examine structures and processes, with a view to improving outcome, that outcome being the quality of care. Most of the approaches covered include the use of standards, and some of the organisations concerned consulted service users, carers, professionals, service providers, or other key organisations or individuals with an interest in the field, in developing the standards. Various methods were adopted to assess compliance with the standards, including observations, interviews, medical record and documentation review.

CHAPTER 17

Standards

The New Oxford Dictionary of English (Pearsall 1998) defines the noun 'standard' as follows:

- a level of quality or attainment
  - a required or agreed level of quality or attainment
  - a grade of proficiency tested by examination or the form/class preparing pupils for such a grade
- an idea or thing used as a measure, norm, or model in comparative evaluations.

Documents used as tools to guide reviewers or assessors when they carry out an external evaluation of an organisation often comprise standards, each being accompanied by criteria, some or all of which need to be fulfilled for the standard to be met. This was the format used in the Health Advisory Service standards (Health Advisory Service 2000, 1999), which are discussed in this book. In practice, the words 'standard', 'criteria' and other connected words and phrases are sometimes used flexibly.

In discussing 'criteria', Donabedian, whilst aware that common usage of this word, and the various associated words and phrases, detracted somewhat from accuracy in their use, chose ideally to define these as 'the phenomena that one counts or measures in order to assess the quality of care' (Donabedian 1982).

He considered that, among the options to be considered in the formulation of criteria in assessing quality, was the choice of an approach to assessment. Accordingly, the criteria would pertain to structure, to process, to outcome, or to a mix of these.

Accreditation (*see* Chapter 18) has been one of the main mechanisms for evaluating quality in healthcare, in the USA, Canada, Australia, the UK and, more recently, in European and other countries worldwide. Common to all accreditation systems is a published set of standards and criteria for assessment of the environment in which clinical care is delivered (rather than clinical practice). These usually derive from a variety of sources including those shown in Table 17.1.

Not all standards used to evaluate healthcare have their origins in that field. In Western European countries, in addition to accreditation, the other evaluation systems mainly used are the International Organization for Standardization (ISO) standards, the European Foundation for Quality Management (EFQM) model and *visitatie*. (These approaches are described in Chapter 19.) All four systems are centred on standards. Accreditation and *visitatie* standards grew from within healthcare, and both these types of standards recognise the uniqueness of healthcare structures, processes and outcomes. ISO and EFQM standards, however, grew

Table 17.1: Sources of standards and criteria for accreditation systems

Sources and inspirations	Examples
Legal regulation	environmental, occupational health; plant safety; employment law
Government guidance etc.	public health policy
National reviews, reports, recommendations	annual reports (e.g. consumer, insurance organisations); national enquiries; formal professional guidelines
Standards from elsewhere	grey literature (e.g. individual hospitals, services); international (e.g. JCAHO, CCHA, ACHS); European collaboration
Research	biomedical, health service
Public expectation	local needs, purchaser requirements
Professional consensus	what practitioners and providers think; expert opinion
Current practice	what actually happens; empirical norms

ACHS = Australian Council on Healthcare Standards; CCHA = Canadian Council on Hospital Accreditation; JCAHO = Joint Commission on Accreditation of Healthcare Organizations (USA). Shaw C (1997) Accreditation Standards in Europe. *Journal d' Économie Médicale*. T15, no.6: 411–17.

from business and industry, and are therefore more global. ISO standards involve an internationally agreed template of standards which is then adopted and modified to meet the needs of each individual country. Business excellence standards, like those of EFQM, are nationally determined, but resemble each other from country to country in both approach and scope. All standards, however, regardless of their origins, grew from the need for comparison and the need to demonstrate quality. To ensure credibility, all these four forms of evaluation have extensive and complex processes for the formulation of standards and their maintenance. In each case, too, there has eventually been the need to make these standards recognisable internationally (Heidemann 2000).

A Royal College of Nursing working party on standards of nursing care emphasised that, in order to be effective and acceptable, standards must be formulated by the professionals themselves and must be explicitly stated. The medical professions have sometimes taken the initiative in setting explicit standards for clinical organisation, as in the cases of Australia and North America, where they co-operated with nursing, administrative and other professional organisations in doing so. The multidisciplinary approach is important, since most aspects of health overlap more than one professional group (Shaw 1982). Current thinking would also place other interested parties, especially service users and carers, amongst those who should be involved in developing standards.

The validity of standards and the reliability of the assessment in which they are utilised are crucial for consistency of the approach used, both within and between the organisations that are evaluated (Shaw 2000); validity and reliability are discussed in Chapters 25 to 27.

CHAPTER 18

Accreditation

Background

The term 'accreditation' (applied to organisations rather than to specialty clinical training) reflects the origins of systematic assessment of hospitals against explicit standards; it developed in the USA from 1917 as a mechanism for recognition of training posts in surgery. That model was the beginning of the Joint Commission on the Accreditation of Healthcare Organizations (JCAHO), was exported via Canada to Australia in the 1970s and arrived in Europe in the 1980s. It is most evident in the UK, Spain, Portugal, The Netherlands, Finland and, by statute, in Italy and France; it was developed in Switzerland (by the Swiss Society for Quality in Health Care) and Germany (jointly by the Medical Chamber and insurance companies). Assessment is by a multidisciplinary team of health professionals against published standards. 'Accreditation', having acquired three different meanings, causes some confusion. Each meaning is correct in its own context (*see* Table 18.1); users need to be aware of the difference between contexts (Shaw 2000).

In this chapter, much of the discussion relates to the second of the definitions given in the table; in addition, some attention is also paid to the third.

All accreditation systems (within the second definition) have explicit standards for organisation against which the participating hospital or service assesses itself before a structured visit by outside 'surveyors', who submit a written report back to

Table 18.1: Meanings of 'accreditation' as used by different professional groups and constituencies

Used by	Intended meaning	Since
Professional bodies	Recognition of specialty training	19th century
Consortia of clinicians and managers	Recognition of service delivery	c1920
International Organization for Standardization	Recognition of agency competent to certificate healthcare providers	1946

Shaw C (2000) External quality mechanisms for health care: summary of the ExPeRT project on visitatie, accreditation, EFQM and ISO assessment in European union countries. *International Journal for Quality in Health Care.* **12**(3): 169–75. Reproduced with permission.

the hospital or service, with commendations and recommendations, for development prior to a follow-up survey. Accreditation may be awarded for a fixed term, or may be withheld by an independent assessment board if the hospital or service does not meet a defined threshold of standards.

One common characteristic of accreditation systems around the world is that, in principle, they are independent of purchasers, providers and government, and participation is voluntary. In practice many agencies influence programmes, either directly or via inducements and sanctions, for example as conditions for licensing or instance reimbursement (Shaw 1997). Several accreditation programmes started out by focusing on hospitals, and subsequently extended their activities to cover other types of healthcare settings. A patient-centred approach was adopted in some schemes.

Below is a summary of programmes in the USA, Canada, Australia and the UK, which have all been in existence for some time. In the UK, the term 'organisational audit' has also been used to describe accreditation. Where the programmes cover aspects relating to mental health services for older people, these are included.

USA

Joint Commission on Accreditation of Healthcare Organizations

In 1917 the American College of Surgeons established the Hospital Standardization Programme. This programme, as originally conceived, was one of the means by which the American medical elite asserted its claim to control the system in which its members worked. The standards devised were directed at creating an environment in which doctors could practise their craft. By 1949, over half the hospitals in the United States were involved. The whole cost of the programme was borne by the College from its membership fees, and it was felt to be too expensive for the College to carry on its own. In 1950, the College approached the College of Physicians and the American Hospitals Association and other bodies to join them to create the Joint Commission on Accreditation of Hospitals (Scrivens 1995a). The Joint Commission was thus founded in 1951. In 1988, it was re-named the Joint Commission on Accreditation of Healthcare Organizations (JCAHO). In 1997, the Joint Commission evaluated and accredited over 15 000 healthcare organisations in the United States, nearly 5 300 hospitals and over 10 000 other healthcare organisations that provided home care, long-term care, behavioural healthcare, laboratory and ambulatory care services. The JCAHO, an independent, not-for-profit organisation, was, at the end of the 1990s, the USA's oldest and largest standard-setting and accreditation body in healthcare.

During a JCAHO survey, a surveyor evaluated the organisation's level of compliance with applicable standards. The surveyor assessed standards compliance in a variety of ways, including observations, interviews, medical record review and documentation review, and used a five-point scale to indicate the organisation's level of compliance with each standard. Once an organisation had received an accreditation award, it was valid for a period of three years, unless revoked for cause.

With regard to mental health services for older people, some such services were included in the Commission's Long Term Care Accreditation Program, which provided accreditation to long-term care organisations from 1966. By 1997, it accredited over 1300 long-term care organisations. It also accredited and provided special accreditation certificates for subacute care programmes and dementia special care units. Long-term care organisations with dementia special care units had to comply with both the regular long-term care standards and intent statements, and the particular intent statements for dementia special care units, which were included in the 1996 Comprehensive Accreditation Manual for Long Term Care (Joint Commission on Accreditation of Healthcare Organizations 1997).

Users of accreditation

As described above, the JCAHO was originally dominated by the medical profession, and its accreditation system appeared to be a model of self-regulation by the healthcare industry. However, it was forced to adapt to changes brought about in the 1960s by the introduction of Medicare and Medicaid (*see* Chapter 8). This, in effect, made hospitals dependent on revenue from tax-financed patients. Public finance brought about a threat of public regulation: the reimbursement of Medicare patients was made dependent on hospitals meeting the federal conditions, enforced by the states, for participation. In effect the state was determining hospital standards. If the JCAHO was to head off the threat of a federal inspectorate – and with it, a threat to its own survival – it had to adapt. A compromise was negotiated. Hospitals accredited by the JCAHO were given 'deemed status', that is, they were deemed to have met the conditions necessary for participation in Medicare.

With deemed status, healthcare organisations were joined by new users of accreditation: the federal government and, later, state governments. In 1995, of the approximately 7000 hospitals meeting the conditions for deemed status for Medicare, about 77% per cent did so through the JCAHO accreditation programme. In 2000, 45 state governments used accreditation in licensing hospitals. In principle, then, the two major characteristics of an accreditation system, as opposed to a system of state regulation, have been maintained: the body defining and monitoring standards remains independent, and participation in the scheme is voluntary. In practice, both principles have been blurred.

By purchasing health insurance for their employees, employers were the principal non-government funders of healthcare in the USA. In the 1980s, as the rising costs of this insurance became a threat to global competitiveness for US businesses, some employers and many insurance companies began making these purchases based on value, i.e. cost and quality (reflected in accreditation). Their demand for cost control also led to new payment mechanisms that capped the amount paid per patient or condition, forcing healthcare organisations to seek efficiencies in care delivery.

Further, employees began contributing to their employer-funded insurance premiums and paying copayments when receiving care. Becoming price conscious, but also worrying about the effects of cost cutting on the quality of care, they too became 'users' of accreditation to help choose among health plans and provider organisations based on value. In addition, with the growth of consumerism in healthcare, patients and their families began to demand more involvement in decision making about their care, including where to get care. Accreditation became a source of information that consumers could use in this decision making (Scrivens 1995a; Schyve 2000).

User impact on accreditation

If the public and its government were to rely on accreditation, it wanted to have its perspective heard in setting policy and standards for accreditation. The JCAHO responded in 1982 by adding public members to its governing board. In 1999, a Public Advisory Group on Healthcare Quality was formed to advise the board on policy issues. Members of the public also expected the JCAHO to respond to their quality-related concerns about accredited organisations. Therefore, it created an Office of Quality Monitoring with a toll-free number that the public could call with their complaints.

The JCAHO met an increasing demand for public accountability of healthcare providers, which stemmed from concerns about both the cost and quality of care. It did this, from 1994, by publicly disclosing, in addition to the accredited organisation's accreditation status, a performance report on each organisation. This report included performance on each of the major foci of the standards (for example respect for patient rights, medication use, infection control), the area(s) in which it received recommendations for improvements, and national comparisons to similar organisations, and from 1997 these reports were placed on the JCAHO's website.

There were increased concerns about the safety of care, driven both by media coverage of adverse events and by growing professional recognition of the frequency of their occurrence. Concern about the frequency of serious adverse events ('sentinel events') led the JCAHO to develop a policy on such events, and accreditation standards for how the healthcare organisation and the Commission should respond when one occurred. The policy was designed to build a national database of sentinel events, and results of analyses, as an educational resource.

The JCAHO responded to the desire to decrease healthcare costs. In 1994–95, all the standards manuals were revised to focus on those activities that were believed to be most associated with the safety and quality of care, to introduce the principles of continuous quality improvement, to be patient centred, and to be performance based (i.e. focused on the goals of key processes, rather than specifying how the goals were to be achieved). It was considered that these revisions gave healthcare organisations the freedom to be innovative in improving efficiency while improving the quality of care.

In addition, in 1997 the JCAHO began developing co-operative agreements with other USA accrediting bodies. Under this programme, an organisation that had a care delivery component accredited by another accreditor need not have the component re-evaluated when the Commission accredited the parent organisation. This policy reduced both cost and duplication of effort for the healthcare organisation.

The JCAHO evolved a complex system of checks and balances. The results from the surveyors were checked by teams of trained staff for consistency and accuracy. Scores derived from the assessment of compliance were aggregated into a decision grid which was then analysed using complex decision algorithms that enabled a final score to be calculated. None of the other accreditation systems had at this stage evolved such a complex procedure to justify their decisions. This could be explained as part of the cultural approach of the USA. It was likely to be due to the two obvious differences between the USA states and other healthcare systems in which accreditation operated: first, that final grading became part of the process for allocating public funds and therefore created a highly defensive attitude on the part of surveyed organisations, second, that many USA hospitals operated (and competed) in a market. A hospital could require a successful review from the JCAHO in order to obtain not only its Medicare and Medicaid allocations, but also to treat patients from the major insurance companies. Without it, the result would be financially disastrous (Scrivens 1995a; Schyve 2000).

Response to market forces

The JCAHO's evolving strategy during the 1980s could be understood as the response of any large institution to challenges or threats in its market position in a changing environment. The JCAHO was in a position of near monopoly for many years. However, as it extended its reach into other areas, such as home care, it faced competition which caused it to change the basis of its accreditation approach. For example, the Community Health Accreditation Program (CHAP), developed by the National League for Nursing, operated under a different philosophy. Whereas the JCAHO had three-yearly, pre-planned visits, and disclosed its findings only to the hospital surveyed, the CHAP had annual unannounced visits, and provided for disclosure of information on its findings. Some of the organisations that supported the CHAP in preference to the JCAHO, charged that the JCAHO had an unfair marketing advantage through its practices. In response, the JCAHO agreed to move to some (5%) annual visits without advance notice and to submit its accreditation findings to Health Care Financing Administration.

As the external agencies were demanding a different approach, the JCAHO was forced to respond to meet their needs. It extended its scope: it widened its accreditation activities to cover not only long-term care, ambulatory facilities and home care, but also agencies that co-ordinated care, referred to as networks. A healthcare network was an entity that directly provided, or provided for, integrated health services to a defined population. A network could offer comprehensive or specialty services. It had to have a central structure which co-ordinated service delivery. The types of organisation covered by the definition of a network were health maintenance organisations (HMOs) (*see* Chapter 8), preferred provider organisations, physicians and hospital organisations, and specialty networks that offered services to HMOs, such as mental health services, and government systems which covered, for example, veterans (Scrivens 1995a; Schyve 2000).

Canada

Canadian Council on Health Services Accreditation

The Canadian Commission on Hospital Accreditation was established in 1953, and in 1958 the Canadian Council on Hospital Accreditation was incorporated. Its purpose was to set standards for Canadian hospitals and evaluate compliance with them. Its accreditation programme was voluntary, free from government intervention, national, bilingual, and not-for-profit. The programme grew in popularity: in 1960, there were fewer than 350 accredited hospitals in Canada; by 1988 the number of accredited facilities approached 1300. Accreditation of mental hospitals began in 1964, and of long-term care in 1978. In 1980, the Canadian Long Term Care Association (subsequently re-named the Canadian Association for Community Care) joined the Council's board of directors.

In 1995, the Council changed its name to the Canadian Council on Health Services Accreditation (CCHSA). An accreditation programme for comprehensive (regionalised) health services was launched, and accreditation of community health services began. Accreditation of home care services commenced in 1996. The mission of the CCHSA was to promote excellence in the provision of quality healthcare and the efficient use of resources in healthcare organisations throughout Canada. In March 1998, 1495 health service organisations were accredited by the CCHSA, and in 1999, the CCHSA had recruited and trained approximately 300 surveyors, from a variety of health professions, to act on its behalf on an honorarium basis. National standards were developed through consultation with the healthcare community. The standards likely to be relevant to mental health services for older people included those relating to long-term care and continuing care organisations, comprehensive health services, mental health organisations, community health services and home care organisations.

The client-centred accreditation programme was based on a philosophy of quality improvement and focused on:

- clients, patients, residents and their families as they went through an episode of care
- the roles, responsibilities and competencies of the professional and support staff as caregivers and team members
- the infrastructure and support services that facilitated the provision of quality client, patient and resident care
- the improvements in the quality of care and services provided.

During the on-site accreditation visit, a team of surveyors met with representative groups from various parts of the health service organisation to discuss the processes of care and support function within the organisation, and the quality improvement initiatives related to them. The survey team met the board of directors, senior administrators, care teams and other supporting teams, such as human resources, environment and information management. Clients and their families were interviewed about their understanding of the care received, their feelings about the quality of care and service, and their level of understanding of their role in the care and treatment process. The survey team also reviewed documentation, and visited key work areas.

Following accreditation, the CCHSA resurveyed the organisation every three years, or conducted focused visits according to the organisation's level of compliance with the standards at the time of their last survey.

The standards of *The AIM Program: achieving improved measurement, the council's accreditation programme for the year 2000*, were based on a population health philosophy. Population health was defined as an approach to planning and managing health services. For health services organisations being accredited with the AIM Program, they were asked if they were accepting and using the determinants of health, integrating their services into the continuum, promoting health and wellness, encouraging community involvement and partnerships, and relying on evidence-based decision making. Pilot test sites that were likely to be relevant to mental health services for older people included those in long-term care, mental health, community health and home care (Canadian Council on Health Services Accreditation 1998a, 1998b, 1999a, 1999b, 1999c).

Features of the Canadian system

There was no Canadian equivalent to the financial incentives to meet standards provided by Medicare in the USA. Its emphasis continued to be organisational education and self-development. The client for accreditation in Canada was the individual healthcare provider. The accreditation process was designed to act as a yardstick by which healthcare organisations could measure their own performance against national standards. However, the Canadian Council permitted some moves towards regulation, at least for training purposes, in that it was a requirement for hospitals wishing to train medical interns and other health professionals and to undertake therapeutic abortions.

The Canadian system differed from the American model in some important respects. It was less bureaucratic and legalistic, and the accreditation documentation was much less complex. There was much less emphasis on trying to reduce the discretion of surveyors by elaborate scoring systems. The surveyors – usually a doctor, a nurse and an administrator – were senior professionals currently working in the healthcare field. The Canadian system was therefore much nearer to a professional peer review model than the American original (Scrivens *et al.* 1995).

The Canadian Council was forced to respond to major reforms implemented within the Canadian healthcare system. Eight of the 10 provinces chose to create regional health boards, with responsibilities for planning and co-ordinating health services and administering the regional health budget. The regions interpreted their responsibilities for healthcare very differently, so that some included within their remit more types of healthcare than others. These changes necessitated a revision of the approach to accreditation followed by the Canadian Council. The basic unit of accreditation was no longer the health service organisation, but accreditation was focused on providing a region-wide review of services. This necessitated the development of new standards, which addressed the interrelationships of care referred to by the Canadian Council as comprehensive health services (Scrivens 1995b).

Australia

The Australian Council on Health Care Standards

In Australia, the initial impetus for accreditation came jointly from the New South Wales branch of the Australian Medical Association (AMA) and the Hospital Association of the adjacent State of Victoria, both of whom had for some years, since the early 1960s, been working independently, and not very successfully, to develop a professional non-governmental organisation to promote standards in hospitals. In 1973 a federal grant supported the appointment of a full-time executive officer. What became the Australian Council on Hospital Standards made a slow start. Some critics said that government interest in hospitals already promoted uniform standards, that the public (unlike in North America) had little freedom to choose which hospital they attended, and that the hospitals had very limited resources to upgrade their services anyway. Furthermore, the state health authorities, which had statutory responsibility for hospitals, viewed with suspicion an organisation that looked as if it intended to tell their hospitals what they should be doing. Thus, the Australian Council on Hospital Standards (later renamed the Australian Council on Health Care Standards, ACHS), which started in Victoria in 1974, although it subsequently extended its role to other states, in 1980 did not include Tasmania or Western Australia. It was an independent body, based on the North American joint commission accreditation model. Like its North American counterpart, the Australian Council adapted its processes over the years. It put much emphasis on reviewing the quality assurance activities of the facilities being accredited, as part of its focus on promoting continuing improvement in the quality of care delivered. In co-operation with the medical colleges, it developed a set of clinical indicators (Shaw 1982; Scrivens *et al.* 1995).

The Australian Council followed a similar path to Canada, in that it moved the focus of standards away from a traditional department-by-department review to what was described as a more dynamic form, addressing the processes that affected an individual patient from the time of admission to the hospital, through treatment, evaluation and follow up (Scrivens 1995b).

United Kingdom

In the early 1990s there were two complementary schemes in Britain, which applied the accreditation, or organisational audit, approach throughout the hospital: the King's Fund Organisational Audit (KFOA) Programme (acute general hospitals) and the South Western Hospital Accreditation Programme (small community hospitals; this scheme subsequently became the Hospital Accreditation Programme, HAP). These had what were perceived to be the principal characteristics of accreditation programmes in North America and Australia at that time:

- independence from funding agencies and operators
- published multidisciplinary standards
- voluntary participation
- preparatory self-assessment phase
- assessment by visiting peer group
- verbal and written feedback to participants
- cycle repeating in one or two years
- support network for participants.

The Hospital Accreditation Programme

The HAP was originally set up in 1990 as a pilot scheme to assess and develop community hospitals in the South Western Region. This was then available throughout the UK from April 1993. The initial standards used were published in 1988 in *Towards Good Practice in Small Hospitals* by the National Association of Health Authorities. They were based on the systematic observation of organisational practices in 54 small hospitals and had been broadly endorsed by 17 national bodies, including seven royal colleges. The standards measured purpose and scope of service, management arrangements, equipment and facilities, operational policies, and personnel and training (Shaw and Collins 1995).

During the first year, 20 hospitals took part. The programme's original objectives were to enhance the effectiveness of community hospitals in the South Western Region, to spread good organisational practices throughout the region, and to develop the principles and practice of health service accreditation in community hospitals in the south west. These aims reflected the nature of community hospitals (defined as being run primarily by general practitioners (GPs) and having no resident medical staff) in Britain, and of the South Western Region, which was geographically widespread, and contained three million inhabitants and 70 small hospitals (Shaw and Brooks 1991). In 2000, since the programme began in 1990, 270 survey visits had been undertaken in 140 organisations. Historically the HAP focused on hospitals with fewer than 200 beds, but in 1999, the programme expanded to include accreditation for community services (Hospital Accreditation Programme 2000).

King's Fund Organisational Audit and The Health Quality Service

A partial accreditation system was developed by the King Edward's Hospital Fund for London, an independent foundation whose mission was to improve the quality of management in the NHS. This scheme evolved from an interest in the experience of other countries with accreditation. In the early 1980s it sent a multidisciplinary team to look at the Joint Commission system in the USA, and the Joint Commission standards were subsequently tried out by two pilot hospitals. Later the fund set up the King's Fund Organisational Audit (KFOA) scheme, whose design was based upon that of Australia: a scheme which, although it incorporated advice from the medical profession and colleagues, was not dominated by them. The original emphasis was on self-improvement: on professional peers learning from each other during the surveying process. Like the systems in other countries, the King's Fund responded to the health service market and widened its scope, by producing standards for community hospitals, primary care and general practice (Scrivens *et al.* 1995).

The Organisational Audit Programme, London, published a draft manual, including standards, in 1989. The growth of the programme was rapid, as the number of hospitals requesting participation increased. Twenty-five units were surveyed in 1991. The KFOA accreditation scheme was launched in April 1995, and by November 1997, 86 NHS hospital trusts and independent hospitals had achieved full accreditation. The KFOA was based on self-regulation and external peer review, using explicit standards and criteria, and rigorously testing compliance. The KFOA offered nationally established standards, but the survey managers who facilitated the accreditation process also helped staff in each NHS trust that took part to implement the standards according to local needs.

Seven elements of good institutional performance, relating to patient focus, were identified: professional practice and effectiveness, personal service, risk management, care environment, access to care, staff training and development, and efficient use of resources. These could be quality assured by establishing relevant national and local standards of good practice, producing appropriate policies, procedures and systems to enable consistent application, and using regular patient-focused performance indicators and information to review results.

It was suggested that many NHS trusts chose the KFOA accreditation scheme because they could measure their performance against nationally established standards. The nearest equivalent at that time was ISO 9002, the international standard for quality management systems (ISO: the International Organization for Standardization, is described in Chapter 19). For ISO accreditation, trusts set their own standards in isolation, and the assessors could come from a manufacturing rather than a specialist healthcare background.

For full accreditation, an organisation had to achieve all 1000+ A-weighted criteria. Of the 86 trusts and independent hospitals that had been accredited by 1997, only three achieved full accreditation at the first attempt. Organisations that were provisionally accredited either submitted further documentation or underwent a 'focused revisit', which tackled those A-weighted criteria that were not achieved first time round. Provisional accreditation was rarely regarded as a failure, but as a motivation to participants to 'go the extra distance'. In the late 1990s, the KFOA was the main institutional level accreditation scheme for healthcare organisations in the UK (Shaw and Brooks 1991; Vidall 1998). At that time, its role was taken over by the Health Quality Service (HQS). The HQS programme could be used by any health organisation, including NHS trusts, health authorities, general practices, nursing homes and independent hospitals. The HQS used standards, self-assessment, service development, peer review, report and (for acute and community services) accreditation (Health Quality Service 1999).

CHAPTER 19

Other external quality improvement mechanisms in Western European countries

Introduction

The main external quality mechanisms used in Western European Union countries are accreditation, *visitatie*, the EFQM model and the ISO series of standards (Shaw 2000). Accreditation is described in Chapter 18; the other three approaches, all of which use standards, are outlined here.

Visitatie

This systematic form of external peer review has become especially popular in the Netherlands where, since the second half of the 1980s, all 28 scientific societies of medical specialists have developed programmes. The programme consists of a systematic site visit by selected peers, who are mostly clinical and often unidisciplinary, leading to an assessment report. Visitation, *visitatie* in Dutch, is organised by specialty and the whole model is inspired by the *visitatie* model for teaching hospitals that has been operational as part of quality assurance in specialty training since 1967. The programmes have their roots in the profession and are developed and executed by the profession. Emphasis is on clinical performance in terms of knowledge, skills and attitude. The various programmes have not conceptualised the healthcare organisation in a coherent way, but take the functioning of a group of specialists in a partnership as the starting point. Over the years the programmes have been systematised and organisational issues, professional development and service quality have been included. However, the functioning as a group of medical specialists of the same specialty within the context of a hospital is the dominant perspective. Standards tend to be derived implicitly from practice guidelines and personal experience. Reports are not available to the public (Klazinga 2000; Shaw 2000).

European Foundation for Quality Management (EFQM)

The EFQM was founded in 1988 by the presidents of 14 major European companies, with the endorsement of the European Commission. The main aim of the

EFQM is to stimulate and assist organisations throughout Europe to participate in improvement activities, leading ultimately to excellence in customer and employee satisfaction, impact on society and business results. In contrast with the ISO, where the implementation of international norms is the goal, the EFQM does not standardise quality systems, but promotes quality management. The instruments to do this are the Award Scheme (the European Quality Award and various national awards, inspired by the Baldridge Award developed in the USA for improvement of quality in production industries), and the publication of a model that can be used for self-assessment. The EFQM model is generic, and is not adapted to specific branches of industry such as healthcare.

Healthcare providers who seek voluntary development or a European Quality Award are assessed against performance standards for service industries in specific areas such as clinical results, patient satisfaction, administration and staff management. Several countries, particularly in Scandinavia, have introduced their own national awards based on the European framework.

In 1997 the Steering Group for model development was established to develop a proposal for an improved EFQM model. The improved model was tested and reviewed by more than 500 model users in Europe, prior to the presentation of the EFQM Excellence model in 1999 at the EFQM representatives' meeting in Geneva, where it was accepted as the approach for subsequent years. The 1999 approach was more focused on results, performance, customers and stakeholders.

The essence of the EFQM approach is a model with nine criteria, which are: leadership, people, policy and strategy, partnership and resources, processes, people results, customer results, society results and key performance results. The nine criteria are grouped in 'enabler' and 'result' criteria. The enablers cover the process, the structure and the means of an organisation. The result criteria cover the aspects of performance in a broad way. The EFQM model is based on the premise that enablers direct and drive the results. Simplified, it means that an organisation with well-developed enablers will have excellent results. The most important result criteria are customer results and key performance results. The most important enablers are processes and leadership.

The EFQM approach is applied in three ways: as a frame of reference for the quality management of an organisation, as a self-assessment tool, and the criteria of the model can be used for the national or European Quality Awards. As a frame of reference for quality management, following a decision by the leaders of the organisation, in most cases a broad training programme is undertaken, to introduce the EFQM way of thinking. Eventually, overall quality policy and specific quality improvement projects are aligned to the nine criteria of the EFQM model and benchmarking and assessments are carried out. Where self-assessment is chosen, in most cases a facilitator or an internal or external consultant prepares and conducts the self-assessment together with the management. The nine criteria and the measuring system are used as the tool to identify the strong and weak points of the quality management of the organisation.

In general, the conclusion by commentators is that the EFQM approach provides a broader and more generic framework than most traditional healthcare approaches. Being generic, it does not go into specific standards and norms for healthcare, as the European accreditation systems such as the KFOA in the UK, or the JCAHO in North America. The EFQM approach is general and aligns conceptually with the ideas formulated by Donabedian (1980, 1982), who looked at the healthcare service as a whole and distinguished between structure, process and outcome quality. The dimensions of structure, process and outcome fit well with the dimensions of the EFQM model. Its attributes (high face validity, self-assessment facilitating experimentation, simplicity and compatibility with the structure–process–outcome approach) help explain its relative popularity in healthcare systems in Western Europe.

In almost all European countries the EFQM approach is used by healthcare organisations for self-assessment. Inpatient and outpatient services, acute care and rehabilitation clinics, specialised and primary care services have used the approach. However, only in the UK and The Netherlands is a national institute formally supporting the practical work (The British Quality Foundation and the Dutch Quality Institute). Other European countries also have quality awards, but in most cases they are not directly related to the EFQM approach. Many institutions take their own responsibility for quality management, use the generic EFQM model, and adapt the subcriteria to their own needs. This is completely in line with the fundamental principles of the EFQM: the work is not directed or structured by a European agency, but is an evolving process (Klazinga 2000; Nabitz *et al.* 2000; Shaw 2000).

International Organization for Standardization (ISO)

The ISO 9000 series is a set of five individual but related international standards on quality management and quality assurance; they are generic and not specific to any particular products. The actual audits are performed by certifying organisations, who mostly operate on a for-profit basis and are recognised by national accreditation councils.

The ISO model mainly conceptualises an organisation in process terms. Like the standards, the model is generic and does not aim to address specific characteristics of a production process, such as whether the product is useful, or the outcomes of the production process. The audit is primarily executed by experts in the ISO norms and not by experts in a particular type of organisation; thus it is not a form of peer review. The justification given for this is that generic norms apply to all types of organisations and the certification relates to the quality system, not the actual content of the work. Applied to healthcare, it helps to strengthen the process orientation of a healthcare service, but will not give any assurance about the appropriateness of the selection of treatments for patients, nor the health outcomes. In general, it does not touch the clinical process, and addresses mainly the managerial processes surrounding clinical decision making. ISO has therefore been used mostly in more mechanical departments, such as laboratories, radiology and transport, although it has also been applied to whole hospitals and clinics. The audit process tests compliance with standards and is not intended in itself for organisational development. In each of the countries concerned, a national body tests and recognises ('accredits') independent agencies as competent to certificate organisations that comply with the standards (Klazinga 2000; Shaw 2000).

Accreditation, *visitatie*, EFQM and ISO in action

Standards

Traditionally, the focus of the standards used reflected the original purpose of the four models: professional performance (*visitatie*), health service delivery (accreditation), management systems (EFQM) and quality systems (ISO). During the 1990s, each moved towards comprehensive standards for organisation, management and clinical performance. For example the revised EFQM model identifies specific domains of results in terms of clinical outcome, and patient and staff satisfaction, and offers a conceptual framework to which standards in other models may be mapped.

Early accreditation programmes used standards based on legislation, expert advice, research, current practice and overseas experience, and expressed them in terms of headings within vertical management units. More recent standards tend to follow patient pathways and emphasise the interface between management units. The development of ISO and EFQM standards is driven by existing users, most of whom are not related to healthcare. *Visitatie* and accreditation standards increasingly emphasise the clinician/management interface, evidence-based medicine and the continuum of care as seen by patients rather than managers (Shaw 2000).

Assessment process

All four models require participants to provide preliminary information and to be able to present selected documents. Some provide a self-assessment questionnaire (ranging from basic data on staff and activity, to a comprehensive checklist of criteria for compliance with standards), and detailed guidance on preparation and external facilitation (typically over 6–12 months) to help the hospital or service towards compliance with the standards. In accreditation, the self-evaluation is commonly the starting point for the external survey team's assessment. With ISO, there is demarcation (absolute in theory, but vague in reality), between the audit and any prior consultancy. Site visits are generally preceded by an external examination of a defined set of internal documents (for example resource and activity data, internal audits, policies and procedures).

The formal external visit (*visitatie*), survey (accreditation), assessment (EFQM) or audit (ISO) lasts from one to five days depending on the size and complexity of the organisation under review, and on the size of the visiting team. ISO focuses on documentation of management systems; the other models include extensive interviews with staff (and sometimes patients), access to management, personnel and patient records, and systematic observation of clinical and support services. In large organisations, observations of topics, staff and sites are based on sampling, on the basis that it is not cost-effective to do otherwise; 'triangulation' (testing of specific issues from several angles or by different observers) is a practical proxy for perfect standards and perfect surveys.

Most models provide a verbal preliminary report, before leaving the site, to test the validity of observations and to ensure that no surprises appear later in the formal written report, which generally includes commendations of positive features as well as noting non-compliance. Recommendations for action on improvement, in order to meet or exceed the standards, are usually provided.

With regard to the surveyors (or visitors, assessors or auditors) competence and credibility are essential attributes of individuals, and each team needs a balance of clinical and managerial expertise, as well as a sound understanding of the standards and assessment process. Selection, training, assessment (and de-selection) of auditors are clearly defined under ISO, but are also systematic under the EFQM and accreditation programmes (which invariably train their own surveyors). Some *visitatie* programmes rely on career experience rather than training (Shaw 2000).

CHAPTER 20

Government-led systems for evaluating health and social services in England and Wales

Evaluating health services: The Commission for Health Improvement

Background

The Commission for Health Improvement (CHI) was established, under the Health Act 1999 and its associated powers, as a non-departmental public body, covering England and Wales, which had statutory powers, but was independent from government. The establishment of the CHI was first announced in the White Paper *The New NHS: modern – dependable* (Secretary of State for Health 1997), where its role was described as '... to support and oversee the quality of clinical services at a local level, and to tackle shortcomings'.

The creation of the CHI was one of a range of measures introduced by the government in the White Paper, to drive quality into all parts of the NHS. They included the setting up of the National Institute for Clinical Excellence (NICE), to lead on clinical and cost-effectiveness, and a system of clinical governance in NHS organisations, to ensure that clinical standards were met. New NHS organisations, primary care groups (PCGs), were created, which gave a more prominent role to local GPs and community nurses, in shaping services for patients (Secretary of State for Health 1997). PCGs could be established at four levels, ranging from, at level one, supporting the health authority in commissioning care, to, at level four, becoming established freestanding bodies, accountable to the health authority for commissioning care, and with the added responsibility for the provision of community health services for their population. Those at levels three and four would become primary care trusts (PCTs) (Secretary of State for Health 1997).

In fact, PCGs were relatively short-lived. PCTs started to be established, in waves, from 2000. In *Shifting the Balance of Power within the NHS: securing delivery* (Department of Health 2001d), the government described a change in role, and reduction in numbers (from 95 to 28), for health authorities, which would become strategic health authorities. Along with this shift was an enhanced role for PCTs, which would become the lead NHS organisations in assessing need, planning and securing all health services and improving health. By April 2002, the new strategic health authorities would be established and new PCTs would be operational.

The CHI's core functions were to:

- provide national leadership to develop and disseminate clinical governance principles
- independently scrutinise local clinical governance arrangements to support, promote and deliver high quality services, through a rolling programme of local reviews of service providers
- undertake a programme of service reviews to monitor national implementation of National Service Frameworks (NSFs, which set national standards and performance measures for specific care groups), and review progress locally on implementation of these frameworks and NICE guidance
- help the NHS identify and tackle serious or persistent clinical problems. The Commission will have the capacity for rapid investigation and intervention to help put these right
- over time, increasingly take on responsibility for overseeing and assisting with external incident inquiries (Department of Health 1998a).

The CHI was to conduct a rolling programme of reviews, visiting every NHS organisation over a period of around three to four years. It was to look for evidence that clinical governance arrangements were working, that they were consistent with established standards, and could develop and sustain services. By 2004, the CHI was to have completed reviews of 500 NHS organisations (Department of Health 1998a).

In April 2002, the Secretary of State for Health announced that the government was to strengthen the system of inspection for health and social services, to ensure clearer public accountability and address the fragmentation in the existing system. An independent, single new Commission for Healthcare Audit and Inspection (CHAI) was proposed, which would bring together the health value for money work of the Audit Commission (see p. 114), the work of the CHI and the private healthcare role of the National Care Standards Commission (*see* p. 118). It was to have responsibility for inspecting both the public and private healthcare sectors. Its principle roles, spelt out in the National Health Service Reform and Health Care Professions Act 2002, were to inspect NHS organisations, recommend special measures where appropriate, set up the Office for Information on Healthcare Performance (responsible for publishing annual comparative NHS performance ratings in England, leading on commissioning national clinical audits and managing annual staff and patient surveys), and publish an annual report on the state of the NHS (Secretary of State for Health 2002; Commission for Health Improvement 2003a, 2003b). When the new organisation commenced operation in April 2004, it branded itself the Healthcare Commission.

Performance ratings for NHS trusts in England, covering the year ended March 2003, were the first to be produced and published by the CHI. The government was responsible for setting priorities, which in turn determined the indicators relating to key targets. Other indicators were designed by the CHI and the Department of Health. The performance ratings system placed NHS trusts in one of four categories, according to which they were awarded from three (top) to zero (bottom) stars. Information from the CHI's clinical governance reviews was used in determining poorly performing and high performing NHS organisations (www. ratings.chi.nhs.uk).

Clinical governance reviews

The CHI's definition of clinical governance was:

> a system of steps and procedures adopted by the NHS to ensure that patients receive the highest possible quality of care. It includes:
> - a patient-centred approach
> - an accountability for quality
> - ensuring high standards and safety
> - improvement in patient services and care (www.chi.nhs.uk).

The CHI commenced a full programme of reviews in NHS acute trusts in 2000. The first reviews of clinical governance in health authorities (including PCGs, local health groups in Wales, and primary care) and trusts providing mental health services commenced in 2000, and the first reviews of clinical governance in PCTs, ambulance trusts and NHS Direct commenced in 2002. The author was employed at the CHI during 2000–2002, and led the development of the methodology for reviewing clinical governance in health authorities and primary care.

The process for reviews, which was streamlined by the CHI following the experience of the initial reviews, was as follows.

Phase 1: The organisation being reviewed collates data, and undertakes planning, including for a staff survey.
Phase 2: The CHI meets and briefs the organisation and a multiprofessional review team carries out the review visit.
Phase 3: The CHI produces a review report; the organisation formulates an action plan, based on findings.
Phase 4: Improvements are delivered, in line with the action plan. Monitoring is undertaken by the strategic health authority (www.chi.nhs.uk).

Evaluating social services: the Social Services Inspectorate and the Audit Commission

The Social Services Inspectorate

The Social Services Inspectorate (SSI) in England was set up in 1985 as a professional division within the Department of Health. The Inspectorate brought professional and management expertise to:

- providing policy advice within the Department of Health
- managing the Department's links with social services Departments and other social care agencies
- inspecting the quality of social care services
- assessing the performance of local councils with social services responsibilities, including 'best value'. (For an account of 'best value', *see* p115.)

The SSI worked through a regional structure; in 2003 there were nine regional offices, each covering the same geographical area as the government office for the region.

The SSI evaluated the quality of local council social services through inspections and through joint reviews with the Audit Commission (*see* p. 114). SSI inspections assessed a specific service area in depth, while joint reviews looked more broadly at how councils performed all of their social services functions and used their resources.

Inspections focused on the quality of services received by users and carers, and the management arrangements for delivering services. Most covered broad service areas, for children and families, child protection, older people, mental health, people with physical or sensory disabilities and people with learning disabilities.

When the SSI inspected, it:

- systematically collected and analysed information from a wide range of sources
- focused on the experience of service users and their carers
- evaluated against standards based on regulations and guidance
- made professional judgements
- provided information to inform the development and implementation of government policy.

From April 2000, the SSI established arrangements to assess systematically the performance of all councils with local social services responsibilities. One of the aims of performance assessment was to ensure that local councils worked effectively with the NHS to address joint health and social care policy and service delivery issues. All local councils were required to complete a delivery and improvement statement each spring, which provided a self-assessment of their progress in delivering against the Department of Health's national objectives and targets, and local improvement plans following inspections and joint reviews. Each year, the SSI brought together evidence from a range of sources about the performance of each local council, to form an overall assessment. This evidence included the provisional performance assessment framework (PAF) indicators, recent inspections and joint reviews, the evaluated delivery and improvement statement, plans submitted to the Department of Health and relevant reports from other inspectorates (Department of Health, Social Services Inspectorate 2000; www.doh.gov.uk/ssi).

In 2002 the Department of Health published the first social services star ratings. These performance ratings were formulated from evidence from published performance indicators, inspection, SSI/Audit Commission joint reviews, review of plans and in year performance information from the SSI and external auditors. These star ratings formed part of local councils' comprehensive performance assessment (*see* p. 116). (www.doh.gov.uk).

In April 2002, the Secretary of State for Health announced that a single inspectorate, the Commission for Social Care Inspection, was to be formed. This was to bring together the work previously undertaken by the SSI, the SSI/Audit Commission Joint Review Team (see below) and the social care functions of the National Care Standards Commission. It was to inspect all social care organisations, public, private and voluntary, assess them against national standards, and publish its findings. It was to register services that needed to meet national standards, inspect and assess the performance of local councils' social services functions, report nationally on social care provision and resource allocation, and provide independent scrutiny of complaints (Secretary of State for Health, 2002; www.doh.gov.uk/ssi/csci.htm).

The Audit Commission

The Audit Commission was established in 1983 to appoint and regulate the external auditors of local authorities in England and Wales, and in 1990 its role was extended to include the NHS. By 1999, its remit covered over 13 000 bodies. The commission operated independently, and derived most of its income from the fees charged to audited bodies. Auditors were appointed from District Audit (a related organisation) and private accountancy firms to monitor public expenditure. Audits ensured that safeguards were in place against fraud and corruption and that local rates were being used for the purposes intended. Auditors assessed expenditure for probity and regularity, and also for value for money. The commission's value-for-money studies examined public services objectively, often from the user's perspective (Audit Commission 1999b).

Joint reviews

Joint reviews, which commenced in the late 1990s, were undertaken on behalf of the SSI and the Audit Commission. An independent assessment was provided of how well the public was served by social services in each council in England and Wales. The review examined how councils organised and delivered services to meet the needs of vulnerable people in their communities.

The SSI/Audit Commission joint review team brought together the expertise of the two organisations to review the performance of all local councils' social services responsibilities. Joint reviews considered how well a council met individuals' needs, shaped services, managed performance and managed resources.

Reviews asked four questions:

1 Are services focused on users?
2 Is the council well placed to shape better services for the future?

3 Is performance managed effectively?

4 Are resources managed to maximise value for money?

Each review drew together the views and experiences of users and carers with evidence about the council's plans, standards and costs, to reach an overall judgement about how well people were served and how well placed the council was to do better in future.

The SSI inspection and SSI/Audit Commission joint review programmes were complementary and scheduled so that each could build on the work of the other (Audit Commission and Department of Health 1998; Audit Commission 1999a; Department of Health 2000).

Evaluating 'best value' in local authorities

'Best value' was announced in the White Paper *Modern Local Government – in touch with the people* (Department of the Environment, Transport and the Regions, 1998). It was described as a duty to deliver services to clear standards, covering both cost and quality, by the most effective, economic and efficient means available. In carrying out this duty, local authorities would be accountable to local people and have a responsibility to central government in its role as representative of the broader national interest. Local authorities were to set standards for all the services for which they were responsible. In those areas such as education and social services, where the government had key responsibilities and commitments, the government itself was to set national standards. Local authorities would need to take the national dimension into account in setting their own standards. Under 'best value', local people would be clear about the standards of services which they could expect to receive, and better able to hold their councils to account for their record in meeting them.

The SSI assessed the performance of local councils with social services responsibilities, in relation to 'best value' in social services. The Audit Commission assessed the performance of local councils relating to 'best value' with respect to all their functions, apart from social services.

The Audit Commission (1999b) publication *A Measure of Success: setting and monitoring local performance targets* was written to help local authorities to respond to the new duty to secure 'best value'. The approach to the use of standards described here was in some respects different from those outlined elsewhere in this book, since here standards, targets and performance measures were to be set by the local council concerned, rather than by the external evaluating body. Local authorities had to report their performance against the Audit Commission indicators each year. They were also required to develop their local indicators and targets as part of a wider process of fundamental performance review and local performance planning (Audit Commission 1999b).

Comprehensive performance assessment (CPA)

The White Paper *Strong Local Leadership: quality public services* (Office of the Deputy Prime Minister 2001) announced a comprehensive and integrated performance framework, with the aim of helping councils deliver better services for their communities. The cornerstone of the framework was comprehensive performance assessments (CPAs), which would provide a clear performance profile for each council. The information would:

- enable a proportionate action plan, linked to the Best Value Performance Plan, to be agreed with each authority to address areas of concern highlighted in the CPA and to help better target resources for support
- inform negotiation of targets and freedoms through local public service agreements (PSAs)
- provide a robust basis for action to tackle poor performance and failure.

Each council's performance and capacity to improve would be assessed, taking into account local circumstances, bringing together:

- performance indicator data (on current performance and past trends)
- Office for Standards in Education (OFSTED), the SSI, the Benefit Fraud Inspectorate and other service-based inspections and assessments together with audit reports
- a corporate governance assessment of the authority as a whole, undertaken in dialogue with the authority and incorporating an element of peer review.

The result would be a 'balanced scorecard' compiled by the Audit Commission with assistance from other inspectorates and bodies with an assessment role, and working with councils themselves. This would identify councils' level of performance. The assessments would be complemented by the performance rating star system for social services. According to the level at which councils were identified to be, flexibilities, freedoms, monitoring and support would be provided.

CHAPTER 21

Towards evaluation of mental health services for older people

Standards to evaluate residential services for older people

Introduction

Standards to evaluate residential services for older people are included here, because many older people in residential services have mental health problems. Such standards, while not specific to them, are relevant to them. The standards described here, and the processes of which they form a part, from the UK and Australia, were intended to be used by the statutory authorities in an enforcement process. In the UK, they were devised as part of a regulatory system; in Australia, sanctions action could be taken against those providers not meeting their obligations, and compliance with the standards was a condition for funding.

United Kingdom

The White Paper *Modernising Social Services* (Secretary of State for Health 1998), set out the government's commitment to improving protection for vulnerable people through new inspection systems and stronger safeguards. Existing regulatory arrangements were considered to be incomplete and patchy, and responsibilities for regulating the various services for adults and children were divided between local authorities, health authorities and the Department of Health centrally. The Registered Homes Act 1984 and its regulations did not set out much detail in terms of the standards that care homes should meet, and there was inconsistency between authorities.

The White Paper proposed the establishment of a new independent regulatory structure, to cover services including residential care homes for adults, nursing homes and domiciliary care provision. The proposals for a new regulatory system, and the national standards, were designed to meet the principles of good regulation outlined in the review of long-term care arrangements carried out by the Better

Regulation Task Force in 1998, which were: transparency, accountability, targeting, consistency and proportionality (Department of Health 1999b).

The proposals in the White Paper were realised in the Care Standards Act 2000, and the explanatory notes accompanying the Act clarified some of its main features (*Care Standards Act 2000: explanatory notes*). The main purpose of the Act was to reform the regulatory system for care services, including residential homes and nursing homes, in England and Wales. For the first time, local authorities were required to meet the same standards as independent sector providers and the new arrangements replaced those set out in the Registered Homes Act 1984.

The Act established a new, independent body for social care and private and voluntary healthcare services in England, the National Care Standards Commission (NCSC). The NCSC, which was to be operational by 1 April 2002, was a non-departmental public body, which would regulate services, including care homes. Provision was made for regulation-making powers to cover the management, staff, premises and conduct of establishments and agencies, and there was also provision for regulations to be made regarding the welfare of service users. The appropriate minister was given the power to publish statements of national minimum standards with which establishments and agencies were expected to comply. Different services were to have different sets of regulations and standards which were to be appropriate to the type of service. The appropriate minister was also given power to make provision as to the conduct of an establishment or agency, including, in relation to independent hospitals and clinics, the arrangements to be made to ensure that any medical or psychiatric treatment or listed services met appropriate standards.

The Act also provided for the Secretary of State to maintain a list of individuals who were considered to be unsuitable to work with vulnerable adults. Individuals employed in care homes, private and voluntary hospitals or clinics, independent medical agencies or NHS establishments, who had regular contact with vulnerable adults in the course of their normal duties, were among the categories that, if necessary, could be considered unsuitable to work with vulnerable adults.

The Centre for Policy on Ageing (CPA) had been commissioned by the government to produce standards for residential and nursing homes for older people. The standards were to be robust, measurable and enforceable, through as full a process of consultation as possible. The CPA established an advisory group, encompassing all the key interests in the field. In addition, they held meetings with providers, regulators and service users, visited homes and reviewed research. Following consultation on the draft standards, the Department of Health published *Care Homes for Older People: national minimum standards* (Department of Health 2001a) (subsequent editions were published in 2002 and 2003). These national minimum standards, which were to apply from 1 April 2002, were core requirements which applied to all care homes providing accommodation and nursing or personal care for older people. They applied to homes for which registration as care homes was required, including residential care and nursing homes which were registered, new facilities, local authority care homes and establishments which had been exempted under the Registered Homes Act 1984.

The standards focused on achievable outcomes for service users, that is, the impact on the individual of the facilities and services of the home. They were grouped under the topics: choice of home, health and personal care, daily life and social activities, complaints and protection, environment, staffing, and management and administration. Each topic was prefaced by a statement of good practice, and each standard was preceded by a statement of the intended outcome for service users to be achieved by the care home.

As mentioned in Chapter 20, in April 2002 the Secretary of State for Health announced that a single inspectorate, the Commission for Social Care Inspection, was to be formed. This was to bring together the work previously undertaken by the SSI (*see* Chapter 20), the SSI/Audit Commission joint review team (*see* Chapter 20) and the social care functions of the NCSC. The new commission was to inspect all social care organisations, public, private and voluntary, assess them against national standards, and publish its findings. It was to register services that needed to meet national standards, inspect and assess the performance of local councils' social services functions, report nationally on social care provision and resource allocation, and provide independent scrutiny of complaints (Secretary of State for Health 2002; www.doh.gov.uk/ssi/csci.htm).

Australia

As discussed in Chapter 13, the government introduced a package of reforms to the aged care system that were based around the unification of the former hostel and nursing home sectors into residential aged care services. The reforms had their legislative underpinning in the Aged Care Act 1997, and its subordinate legislation, the Aged Care Principles, which came into effect on 1 October 1997 (Commonwealth Department of Health and Aged Care: Aged and Community Care 2001).

The Aged Care Standards and Accreditation Agency, an independent body established as part of the reform process, began operation in 1998. Its role was to ensure that residential aged care homes reached high standards of care, through inspecting homes for compliance with residential care standards and supporting them in developing systems for continuous improvement. Accreditation was linked to government funding, and aged care homes that were not accredited did not receive government subsidies.

Accreditation was granted to those aged care homes that were considered to be operating in accordance with the legislative requirements of the Aged Care Act 1997, and providing high quality care within a framework of continuous improvement. All aged care homes were required to meet accreditation requirements by January 2001 to continue to be eligible for Commonwealth government funding. Homes could be accredited by the agency for a period, generally one or three years, depending on how well they were assessed to be performing.

The accreditation standards introduced under the Act were:

- management systems, staffing and organisational development
- health and personal care

- resident lifestyle
- physical environment and safe systems.

For each aspect of each standard, the accreditation process considered homes' policies and procedures, staff practices, resident/carer feedback and other evidence.

Under the Act, aged care homes had to comply with a dimension of quality control specific to aged care, known as certification. This was the process of assessing homes against specified building and care standards. To achieve certification, a residential home was inspected to determine whether it met certain minimum building standards relating to fire safety, security, resident privacy, occupational health and safety, lighting, heating, cooling and ventilation. As an incentive for providers to meet these standards, aged care homes had to be certified in order to be able to charge accommodation payments, and to receive a concessional resident supplement for eligible residents. The certification status of a home was considered and weighted heavily in assessment for accreditation. Where an aged care home failed accreditation, it lost its entitlement to Commonwealth subsidy for all residents on or after 1 January 2001.

With regard to quality of care, under the reforms, this was addressed through several discrete elements, which collectively could be considered a quality assurance framework. This framework comprised the following elements:

- *standards for care*: quality care was defined as being provided when the specific standards of care were met. The standards were specified in the legislation (Aged Care Act 1997 and Quality of Care Principles), were outcome focused and applied to all approved aged care homes. The new standard was designed to encourage aged care homes to have appropriate systems, processes and procedures in place to promote continuous improvement
- *information and education* for stakeholders, provided by The Aged Care Standards and Accreditation Agency
- *assessment and monitoring* undertaken by the agency, to ensure that compliance was ongoing. Systems of spot checks and support visits were also in place
- *feedback mechanisms* based on achievement of outcomes, as experienced by residents and their relatives.

In March 2000, the minister established the Aged Care Accreditation and Compliance Forum, comprising key stakeholders, to look at accreditation and compliance issues as they affected residents, providers and government. Three working groups were initially established to review and advise on certain initiatives and developments. These groups were:

- developing a code of conduct for the industry
- considering medical and pharmaceutical practice in aged care
- considering the development of enhanced aged care qualifications for staff.

The government recognised that there were costs associated with meeting the new standards and that some aged care homes would require assistance in order to remain viable. A technical reference group (TRG) was established in 1997, to explore restructuring issues, and advise on the spending of a $20 million restructuring fund made available by the government in the 1998–99 budget.

Within the new system, sanctions action could be taken against any provider that did not meet responsibilities under the 1997 Act for quality of care, user rights, accountability and the requirements relating to the allocation of places. Under the quality assessment framework, the department had a greatly enhanced capacity to monitor and report on sanctions. The department reported that only a small minority of providers failed to meet their obligations under the Act and were subject to sanctions action.

Standards to evaluate aspects of mental health services for older people

This section describes standards which were developed to evaluate certain aspects of mental health services for older people, but not the full range of services. It does not include The Health Advisory Service (HAS 2000) standards to evaluate mental health services for older people, which cover all aspects of mental health services for older people, and are discussed in depth in Chapters 23 and 24 (Health Advisory Service 2000, 1999).

United Kingdom

Social Services Inspectorate

The Department of Health, Social Services Inspectorate (SSI) (1993) publication, *Inspecting for Quality: standards for the residential care of elderly people with mental disorders* was aimed primarily at those who purchased, registered, inspected or managed the provision of residential services, and was also intended to be useful to staff who worked in residential homes. (For an account of the SSI, *see* Chapter 20.) It was produced by a small group of SSI and Department of Health staff, after consultation with representatives of users and providers in the field. For the purposes of the document, elderly people with mental disorders were defined as people over the age of 65 years who suffered mental health problems, whether these were organic or functional.

The document included a section on 'Issues, problems and good practice' in relation to older people with mental health problems, and made practical suggestions for each of the topics raised. The standards covered the areas of values, decision making, risk taking, restraint, environment, healthcare, relatives and friends, and equal opportunities. Each standards section included criteria, and evidence to look for, to establish whether the standards and criteria were met (Department of Health, Social Services Inspectorate 1993).

The SSI conducted an inspection of services for older people with dementia in the community in eight local authorities between September 1995 and March 1996. The purpose was defined as:

> ... to evaluate arrangements and service provided or purchased by local authorities to maintain older people in the community, including home support, day care and short term breaks. To include the evaluation of independent sector provision where appropriate and relevant and to have regard to collaborative arrangements with health professionals.

Fieldwork was underpinned by a survey of 50 active cases in each authority and analysis of this material informed the report. The methodology included interviews with social services departments, health and independent service managers and practitioners and carers, and visits to sites providing services. Each SSI inspection team was assisted by a senior nurse from an NHS regional office or health trust and by a lay assessor. The inspection used standards and criteria based on legislation, guidance and accepted good practice. They were drawn up by the SSI in consultation with administrative and professional colleagues in the Department of Health and experts from the field. The standards covered the areas: strategies, policies and procedures, accessing services, assessment and management of risk taking, protection from abuse, and equality of opportunity. In addition, a questionnaire was completed by care managers. Findings were reported under the headings of service delivery, strategies and plans, assessment and care planning, monitoring and review, assessment and management of risk taking, protection from abuse, and equality of opportunity. Action points for social services departments were included (Department of Health, Social Services Inspectorate 1996).

Alzheimer's Disease Society

The Alzheimer's Disease Society (the Alzheimer's Society from 1999), a national voluntary organisation, had a Care Consortium, the activities of which included:

- setting standards for day care and home care services run by Society branches, in consultation with carers, professionals and branch representatives
- providing support and advice to its branches in all aspects of planning and delivering quality dementia care
- providing information and training for management committees, staff and volunteers to enable the care services to reach the quality standards
- monitoring the quality of the society's care services as part of a formal quality assurance system.

The standards contained in the document *The Alzheimer's Disease Society Quality Assurance Initiative* (Alzheimer's Disease Society 1996), which were produced by the consortium, were devised to enable the society to achieve consistent high quality in its care services for people with dementia. Consultation was carried out with carers, people with dementia, volunteers and staff. The standards were based on the principles of individualised care, dignity and respect, and understanding and supporting carers. They were grouped in the three areas of client care, staffing, and service management and administration.

The society aimed to introduce the standards to its home care and day care services in England, Wales and Northern Ireland. A monitoring policy and procedure were developed, to be implemented in all the society's care services, and training was to be provided. The consortium set up a care service audit team, whose members were trained to undertake audits of society care services on a national basis (Alzheimer's Disease Society 1996).

World Health Organization

The World Health Organization Division of Mental Health and Prevention of Substance Abuse (1997) publication, *Quality Assurance in Mental Health Care: checklists and glossaries. Volume 2*, contained a *Day Hospitals for the Elderly Mentally Ill Glossary*, which included criteria grouped under the headings of physical environment, administrative arrangements, staffing, admission process, care process, interaction with families, outreach, and discharge and follow up. Beneath each criterion were explanatory details, and, in places, clarification regarding how to rate the criterion (World Health Organization Division of Mental Health and Prevention of Substance Abuse 1997).

The observational method to measure the quality of life for older people in long-stay care

Clark and Bowling (1989) carried out an observational study in order to measure the quality of life of older people in two different types of long-stay care (two NHS nursing homes and a hospital ward). This formed part of a wider evaluation study of these two forms of institutional care. Much research on the institutional care of older people had been positivistic in approach, largely based on survey techniques or extraction of information from records (for example deaths), and assumed that the circumstances of older people could be completely measured using such scientific approaches. It was, however, often difficult to identify objective parameters and measurable criteria with which to evaluate care of older people in institutional settings.

Positivist scales of mental and physical impairment and of life satisfaction were found to be inadequate in terms of discriminating between hospital and nursing home settings. Qualitative techniques could give insights into the behaviours, moods, interactions and atmospheres between settings, which were difficult to measure using traditional methods. The measurement of outcomes, using conventional methods, was still likely to be important to evaluate long-stay care. In order to consider wellbeing, however, patient preferences for inputs to the process should be considered, rather than ultimate outcomes, although feelings about care may be difficult to elicit from an institutionalised population. It appeared that an approach utilising multiple methods was essential in evaluation research, given that a single measure may not be sufficiently sensitive (Clark and Bowling 1989).

The application of a direct observation method which was developed for the assessment of the behaviour of older people with dementia who were long-stay patients (Bowie and Mountain 1993) produced findings which were significant in relation to the quality of care. The method was used to assess the behaviour of patients during their waking day on seven long-stay wards in the Yorkshire Region. The technique recorded behaviour in real time, using portable computers. Behaviour was recorded in seven categories, as shown in Table 21.1.

Table 21.1: Categories for assessing behaviour of older people with dementia who were long-stay patients (Bowie and Mountain 1993)

	Category	Description of behaviours
A	Self-care	Independent participation in activities of daily living – includes eating, drinking, dressing, washing, and purposeful movement
B	Social engagement	Any activity where patient appropriately and actively engaged with their environment – includes participation in social activities, making conversation, reading, and watching television
C	Reception of care	Activities where patient is being treated/cared for by staff and is not displaying independence
D	Motor activity	Unnecessary, often excessive, movement and activity – includes aimless wandering, restlessness, rocking, fidgeting and repetitive movements
E	Antisocial	Behaviours which violate, or cause distress to, others – includes physical and verbal aggression, screaming or shouting, and stealing
F	Inappropriate	Behaviours which would normally be seen as unacceptable, but do not violate others – includes sucking fingers, urinating inappropriately, spitting or throwing food on the floor, and talking to oneself
G	Neutral	Patient is detached from the environment – includes sitting or standing and doing nothing, and sleeping

Bowie P and Mountain G (1993) Using direct observation to record the behaviour of long-stay patients with dementia. *International Journal of Geriatric Psychiatry.* **8**: 857–64. Reproduced with permission.

Observations were made of 110 residents of the wards with a diagnosis of dementia. Almost 114 hours of observed behaviour were recorded. From this it was possible to establish the proportion of the waking day an average patient spent exhibiting each type of behaviour. The results are shown in Table 21.2.

It was noticeable that well over 50% of time was accounted for by neutral behaviour; in other words, for more than 50% of the waking day the patients were doing nothing at all. It could also be seen that on average, patients only received

Table 21.2: Proportion of time spent on each specified category of behaviour by older people with dementia who were long-stay patients (Bowie and Mountain 1993)

	Category	% of time spent
A	Self-care	8.6
B	Social engagement	5.5
C	Reception of care	5.3
D	Motor activity	18.7
E	Antisocial	0.2
F	Inappropriate	11.3
G	Neutral	56.5

Bowie P and Mountain G (1993) Using direct observation to record the behaviour of long-stay patients with dementia. *International Journal of Geriatric Psychiatry.* **8**: 857–64. Reproduced with permission.

care for just over 5% of their waking day; this amounts to an average of 41½ minutes of care per patient during the waking day. The proportion of time spent in constructive behaviours – self-care, social engagement, and receiving care – was at most 19.4% of the waking day. It was likely, however, that this was an over-estimate, as on occasions these behaviours will have occurred concurrently. Over 80% of the day was spent either doing nothing or engaged in useless activity.

The fact that on average these patients only managed self-care activities for less than 10% of the time was probably a reflection of the advanced illness from which they were suffering, although the relative lack of therapeutic activity on these wards may have contributed to an apathetic state in which self-care would be mini-mised. The marked increase in self-care activity at mealtimes, however, suggested that some supervised independence was being encouraged by the staff. The lack of self-care activity from the patients did not appear to have been compensated by large amounts of received care, as on average this amounted to only 5.3% (or 41½ minutes) of the time. This figure appears surprisingly low, but clearly staff had to spend significant periods of time planning care and recording clinical information, and time was also spent supervising patients without giving 'hands-on' care. Whether or not this amount of 'hands-on' care was the most productive use of staff time could not be answered by this study.

The average amount of time that patients were socially engaged was worryingly low, and implied a lack of staff involvement or preoccupation with physical care. Much of the social engagement recorded was between patients and not engagement with members of staff. This lack of engagement could not be excused on the basis of staffing levels, as not infrequently three or more staff would be present in patient areas but conversing among themselves or completing care plans rather than engaging the patients.

It seems, then, that observational techniques, applied in care settings for older people, have a valuable role to play in ascertaining the quality of care.

Evaluation of mental health services for older people in the UK: the Health Advisory Service (HAS)

The HAS prior to 1997

The NHS Hospital Advisory Service, which was established in 1969, covered hospital services for, in the terminology of the times, people who were mentally handicapped, mentally ill, geriatric or chronically sick. Its functions were:

> . . . by constructive criticism and by propagating good practices and new ideas, to help to improve the management of patient care in individual hospitals (excluding matters of individual clinical judgement) and in the hospital service as a whole: and to advise the Secretary of State for Social Services about conditions in hospitals in England and the Secretary of State for Wales about conditions in hospitals in Wales (Department of Health and Social Security/Welsh Office 1971).

The professional staff were recruited on secondment for periods of one or two years. They visited hospitals in teams, normally consisting of five people, drawn from the professional groups: consultant, senior nurse, ward sister or charge nurse, hospital administrator and social worker. Visits, which were initially to long-stay hospitals, were expected to take from a few days to a week to complete, depending on the size of the hospital. The visiting teams were to look at the full range of services, and to consider how far they conformed to norms or minimum standards and other policies recommended regionally or nationally. In particular, the Hospital Advisory Service was to seek information about and, where appropriate, give advice on:

- the service the hospital affords to the community and the links it has with the community
- the organisation of, and channels of communication within, the hospital group including relations between the hospital management committee and staff, and relations between doctors, nurses, administrators and other professions
- relations between staff and patients
- the physical conditions and staff ratios within the hospital (Department of Health and Social Security/Welsh Office 1971).

Despite a considerable number of requests that the Hospital Advisory Service should develop a set of standards that could be applied at all hospitals, it felt that the setting of standards was a matter for the Department of Health and Social Security, and that the visiting team should assess the local hospital in the light of its own professional expertise (National Health Service 1972).

From April 1976 the remit and name of the service changed. It became the Health Advisory Service (HAS), with a responsibility covering not only hospital services but also community health services and the links between the two. In addition, the HAS was to collaborate with the social work services in England and Wales in establishing joint multidisciplinary teams to review together the complementary services provided in an area by health and social services (National Health Service 1976).

By 1984, the purpose of each HAS/SSI visit was described as:

- to look at existing services for the client group concerned
- to provide an objective assessment of those services
- to advise those concerned on how to build constructively on what they have, by concentration on:
  - methods of management and patient care organisation
  - interdisciplinary collaboration
  - education and training of all grades of staff
  - co-operation between agencies, especially in planning
  - mobilisation of the necessary resources (NHS Health Advisory Service 1985).

In reviewing the HAS in 1991, ministers decided that it should continue with its core remit, but that it should be repositioned to enable it to conduct its functions within a reformed NHS. They subsequently decided to extend the HAS's remit to give it explicit responsibilities for monitoring the quality of healthcare and the performance of purchasers. In order to discharge these responsibilities, the HAS developed four main styles of activity: thematic reviews, ministerial reviews, specialist advisory services, and the local review and advisory service. The local review and advisory service provided advice to purchasers and providers at the request of regional health authorities and at the instigation of local services themselves (NHS Health Advisory Service, 1996).

The HAS from 1997 (HAS 2000)

Background

In 1997 the service was reconstituted as the Health Advisory Service (HAS 2000), with management responsibility held by a consortium comprising the Royal College of Psychiatrists, the Royal College of Nursing, the British Geriatrics Society and the Office for Public Management. Representatives of these organisations were joined on the trust board the following year by members of the Association of Directors of Social Services. The organisation's terms of reference included:

> to develop a pro-active advisory and consultancy service with the aims of improving the delivery of health and social care services for mentally ill and older people.

The author was employed at the HAS from 1997 to 2000, and is therefore able to give this account from both organisational literature and personal experience.

The service evaluation framework development programme

To fulfil its remit, HAS 2000 undertook a programme of development work to devise standards, methods and instruments to underpin evaluations of commissioner and provider organisations by teams of external assessors. This was to bring a more thorough, systematic and consistent approach to the traditional 'inspection' role, and support the development of indicators of best practice. The new service evaluation method was piloted in early 1998 and operational by April of that year. The instruments created were used by HAS 2000 to evaluate services in England and Wales. Methodologies and tools were developed for evaluation of health and social care services in the following areas:

- child and adolescent mental health (age group: under 18)
- adult mental health (age group: 18 to 64)
- mental health services for older people (age group: 65 and over)
- mentally disordered offenders
- care of older people (age group: 65 and over).

Methodologies were developed separately for substance misuse, by the Substance Misuse Advisory Service, which formed part of HAS 2000.

In order to ensure consistency of approach in developing the tools and methodologies, and provide support for activities such as literature searches, and agreement on scaling standards, a central team was established, comprising the (then) joint chief executives, the service development advisers (SDAs) (of whom the author was one), the associate director, substance misuse, and a programme manager, employed on a consultancy basis.

For each service area, a specialist team of two people was created, to undertake the development of the evaluation methodologies and tools, consisting of a SDA and an external adviser who was an expert in the client area concerned. The SDAs brought with them a variety of skills and experience, in the fields of service reviews, management, policy and planning. For each client area, an advisory network was established, comprising organisations and individuals with a particular interest in the field.

Standards and criteria in the evaluation instruments were based on information from key documents, extracted using a system of content analysis. For ease of use and consistency, rating of the standards was on a three-point scale, of 'met', 'part met', or 'unmet'. Draft versions of the instruments were revised through consultation and pilot reviews. A technical editor (the author) was seconded within the organisation for six months during 1998–99, to edit the evaluation instruments, to ensure consistency and accuracy. A more detailed account of the methodology used is given in Chapters 23 and 24.

Mental health services for older people

As for all the client groups included in the HAS service evaluation framework development programme, a sub-project was devised for mental health services for older people (MHSFOP). The objectives of the MHSFOP sub-project were:

- to develop comprehensive and robust methodologies and tools for the evaluation of mental health/social care services for older people with mental illness in the target organisations
- to ensure that the HAS is in a position to provide such evaluation services through the use of these validated methodologies and tools by April 1998, having piloted and refined protocols in pilot sites beforehand
- to highlight areas where organisational development is required.

The definition of the client group was people aged over 64 with mental illness. Those on the 'margins' were 'graduates' (those with mental illness who have reached age 65, or over) and those under 65 with dementia.

The development of the Health Advisory Service

In August 2003 the Centre for Mental Health Services Development (CMHSD) merged with the HAS, to form the Health and Social Care Advisory Service (HASCAS). The board of trustees comprised representatives of the Royal College of Psychiatrists, the Royal College of Nursing and the Office for Public Management, together with others. HASCAS, a 'not-for-profit' organisation, offered evidence-based service development to health agencies, government departments, voluntary organisations, probation services and universities. The client groups remained the same as those covered by HAS 2000, with the addition of learning disability and the area of prison health.

Standards were one of the tools used by HASCAS in service development; examples of other mechanisms used were the development of care pathways, and training. When standards were used, they were developed as appropriate for the proposed piece of work. The evidence-based approach included reviewing the literature and talking with practitioners (personal communication, Hilary Rowland 2004).

CHAPTER 22

Comparative analysis of approaches to evaluation

Introduction

In this chapter, a comparative analysis is made of the approaches to evaluating health and social care, and mental health services for older people, which are described in Chapters 18–21. Such a comparative analysis is not straightforward. For some topics relating to the evaluation approaches, information in the literature was covered consistently enough for some analysis to be made; for other topics, however, this was not the case. In order to address this problem, where feasible, key people involved in the various approaches were contacted by post, email or personal contact, using a simple questionnaire, to ask them whether certain key elements were included in the development of the evaluation approach. This exercise, and its findings, are described on pp. 135–7. A comparison is made between the accreditation systems in the Anglophone countries, and commentary is provided on convergence between the four external quality improvement mechanisms in Western European countries, and a comparative analysis is made of all the evaluation mechanisms considered.

Comparison between the accreditation systems in Anglophone countries

In the United States, Canada, Australia and the UK, all the systems of accreditation were similar in the basic approaches and the standards used. (The discussion in this chapter does not include accreditation carried out by Australia's Aged Care Standards and Accreditation Agency, which commenced operation in 1998. This is described in Chapter 18.) There was also convergence between these countries in the way they revised those approaches and standards. All devised or considered outcome indicators which measured the quality of care provided more directly than the traditional review of processes and procedures. The focus shifted increasingly towards assessing quality in terms of the experience of those receiving care. There were, however, some striking differences. In the USA, the JCAHO became a quasi-regulatory body. Accreditation became the key to unlocking access to public funds and as such, virtually indistinguishable from state regulation. In contrast, accreditation in Britain was seen predominantly as an exercise in self-improvement, where it was up to individual providers to decide whether or not to participate. Canada and Australia were somewhere in between. In neither case was accreditation a form of regulation, i.e. a condition for the receipt of public finance (except in the case of Australia's Aged Care Standards and Accreditation Agency: *see* Chapter 18). But in both cases, there was, in contrast to Britain, a national body using national standards which, unlike the USA where the JCAHO faced competition from other agencies, had a monopoly of whole hospital accreditation activities. Even though participation in accreditation remained voluntary in theory, providers risked a certain stigma and possible loss of competitive credibility if they opted out. Therefore, the lines between accreditation and regulation were blurred (Scrivens *et al.* 1995).

In the USA, Canada and Australia, all three accreditation systems adapted their standards and their approach to assessing compliance over the years. In the 1990s they revised their standards to reflect the changing functions of hospitals, seeking to move away from a focus on departments towards one of patient experience of hospital systems. They all moved towards trying to find standards that would reflect the integration of hospital services rather than examining them in isolation (Scrivens 1995a).

Accreditation as a mechanism for external evaluation

Although directed at quality improvement, the process of accreditation was problematic as a tool for assuring quality. The standards were not validated for assuring quality in the production of health; they merely suggested consensus on good organisational practices. The survey process itself presented problems for quality assurance. Surveys permitted snap-shots in time, they did not monitor the continuous delivery of healthcare. In the long periods between surveys, up to four years, compliance with the standards may have deteriorated. Standards were continuously being revised, usually every year. Therefore, a high complying health service provider may have found it was out of step with the new standards when a survey was conducted four years later. Surveys were imprecise mechanisms for assuring comparability and validity. Even the JCAHO, after attempts to ensure surveyor consistency, failed to guarantee lack of surveyor variability. Criticism was directed at the state surveyors, who were found to vary in their judgements, between surveyors, but also across states.

The surveyors' judgements, so crucial to the overall success of accreditation in the minds of the participants, were invariably subjective and biased. There were problems in determining whether truly reliable information about the hospital could be gathered in this way. It was possible to ask whether a hospital had a clear procedure for dealing with budget overspending. But although obtaining answers to questions like these may have helped achieve conformity to set standards, did this process enable assessment of whether a hospital was good or not? A study of the Australian system in 1980 (Duckett 1983) revealed that 46% of the surveyors' recommendations were not tied to a standard. If accreditation was about evaluation of hospital performance, then the surveyors' report was a critical factor. Therefore, the lack of consistency between the report and the framework of standards used to some extent invalidated the process. Accreditation may have been a good tool for encouraging an awareness of quality questions, but whether it was an acceptable process for judging quality of care provided was certainly not proven (Scrivens 1995b, pp. 178–9). Failure to prove a causal link between compliance with process standards and improved clinical results has dogged the development of health service accreditation throughout the world; but if that argued against accreditation it also argued against clinical audit and continuing education (Shaw and Collins 1995).

Issues surrounding the convergence between the four models of evaluation in Western European countries

The four models (*visitatie*, accreditation, EFQM and ISO) have begun to converge. So far this convergence has been spontaneous and opportunistic, rather than planned collaboratively. Given that the models were originally designed for different purposes, complete harmony may be neither feasible nor useful. But clearer demarcation of the scope and contribution of each model could increase efficiency and reduce duplication in the external quality improvement market.

Effective convergence would require developments on a number of fronts. As discussed in Chapter 4, ventures requiring examination of activity across European countries are hampered by lack of comparable information, and differences in concepts of types of healthcare between countries. The ExPeRT project (a European Union project on external peer review), and other initiatives addressing evaluation of healthcare quality on a European or international basis have made a contribution in this regard (Bohigas and Heaton 2000). However, there is still some way to go.

In addition, the following issues would need to be addressed. There is a need for national co-ordination, identifying mechanisms to promote consistency within and between models. In The Netherlands, for example, a council for harmonisation of external quality review in healthcare was set up to recognise and integrate the four models with national policy and legislation; and in the UK a voluntary forum aimed to promote convergence of over 30 accreditation and *visitatie* programmes.

In terms of communication and liaison across Europe, and internationally, adoption of common definitions between models would need to be agreed, especially reconciliation with ISO terminology. International conventions for standards would need to be adopted, consistent with the principles of ISO and EFQM; new programmes would need to be tested against these principles. With regard to assessment, common standards would be needed (for example, those developed by the ALPHA project of The International Society for Quality in Health Care, ISQua) for programme operation, particularly internal mechanisms to minimise observer variation and promote reliability and consistency. In relation to quantification, there would be a need to make explicit the measurement and weightings of compliance with standards as a basis for the evaluation of reports, and for tracking progress of healthcare providers over time and in relation to similar organisations. A common core curriculum of knowledge, attitudes and skills required, and reciprocal training programmes, would need to be developed for assessors (Shaw 2000).

Were these steps to be taken, there would remain potential hurdles to the growing convergence between the models resulting in better healthcare. The existing distribution of responsibilities for quality of care differs among the healthcare systems in Europe. This will affect the implementation of more uniform external quality assurance schemes, as it implies shifts in power and control.

Features of external evaluation that have become important include the involvement of people other than health professionals, patient orientation, patient empowerment and efficiency. These may result in a focus away from clinical decision making and the practice of medicine; some may perceive this as a loss.

All models have the tendency to become bureaucratic, especially when they function for a longer period of time. Should this happen, it would undermine the potential of the models to introduce change and could stifle innovation in healthcare (Klazinga 2000).

Comparison of all the approaches considered

Table 22.1 provides an analysis of features of the approaches to evaluating health and social care examined in this book. All used national standards, except the CHI's clinical governance reviews, joint reviews by the SSI and the Audit Commission, 'best value', the HAS pre-1997, and the observational methods. Of these, the CHI used a review issues document as a basis for collecting evidence, and an assessment framework in order to make assessments on the performance of the NHS organisation being reviewed in relation to each component of clinical governance. joint reviews were based around a set of underlying questions. 'Best value' related to national performance indicators, and standards, targets and performance measures were to be set by local councils. In the observational methods, a defined set of behaviours were observed, and a consistent rating mechanism was used as a measure.

As mentioned in Chapter 21, HAS prior to 1997 considered that it was the role of the Department of Health and Social Security to set standards, and that the visiting team should assess services in the light of their own professional expertise. As stated in Chapter 21, HAS after 1997 in fact undertook its programme of development work to devise standards, methods and instruments to underpin evaluations, to bring a more thorough, systematic and consistent approach to the traditional 'inspection' role. On the basis of the methods examined, therefore, it could be argued that national standards, or similar statements against which services can be measured, are widely accepted as an integral part of mechanisms for evaluating health and social care.

Not surprisingly, as all the accreditation programmes followed a similar model,

Table 22.1: Analysis of approaches to evaluating health and social care

	National standards	Local standards/ flexibility	Specific to MHSFOP	Part of enforcement process
Accreditation				
USA	✓	✗	✗	✗
Canada	✓	✗	✗	✗
Australia	✓	✗	✗	✗
UK: KFOA/HQS	✓	✗	✗	✗
UK: HAP	✓	✗	✗	✗
Other external QI mechanisms in Western European countries				
Visitatie	✓	✗	✗	✗
EFQM	✓	✗	✗	✗
ISO	✓	✗	✗	✗
Standards for residential services for older people				
UK	✓	✓	✗	✓
Australia	✓	✗	✗	✓
Standards for MHSFOP				
UK: SSI	✓	✗	✓	(✓)
UK: HAS from 1997	✓	✗	✓	✗
UK: ADS	✓	✗	✓	✗
Worldwide (WHO)	✓	✗	✓	✗
Evaluating health services in England and Wales				
CHI	✗	✗	✗	✓
Evaluating social services				
SSI	✓	✗	✗	✓
Joint reviews	✗	✗	✗	✓
Best value	✗	✓	✗	✓
HAS pre-1997	✗	✗	✓	✗
Observation				
Clark and Bowling 1989	✗	✗	✗	✗
Bowie and Mountain 1993	✗	✗	✓	✗

MHSFOP	Mental Health Services for Older People	ISO	International Organization for Standardization
KFOA	King's Fund Organisational Audit	CHI	Commission for Health Improvement
HQS	Health Quality Service	SSI	Social Services Inspectorate
HAP	Hospital Accreditation Programme	HAS	Health Advisory Service
QI	Quality improvement	ADS	Alzheimer's Disease Society
EFQM	European Foundation for Quality Improvement	WHO	World Health Organization

they had several common features. All used standards that applied nationally, and did not offer scope for local flexibility. None of the accreditation programmes were specific to mental health services for older people, and none formed part of an enforcement process.

The two sets of standards for residential services for older people both used standards that applied nationally, although the UK scheme allowed local flexibility. Both were part of an enforcement process: in the UK they formed the basis of a regulatory structure, and in Australia compliance was necessary for continued funding, and sanctions could be imposed.

Standards specifically for mental health services for older people showed interesting similarities. All used national standards, and none allowed scope for local flexibility. They were not generally part of an enforcement process, although when the SSI used standards as part of an inspection, this was part of such a process. It should be noted that the SSI and the HAS (from 1997) both, in addition to devising standards for this client group, also used standards for a number of other groups; and that the World Health Organization (WHO) standards, which were in fact criteria, related specifically to day hospitals.

The approaches to evaluating social services departments in general, again, had much in common, as may be expected since the SSI was the, or a, leading player in both. When acting alone, the SSI used standards, although in the joint reviews (SSI and Audit Commission), none were used. There was not scope for local flexibility, and the methods were not specific to mental health services for older people. Both approaches were part of an enforcement process.

'Best value' was part of an enforcement process, in that it was a duty of local authorities, set out in a government White Paper. Prior to 1997, HAS was not part of an enforcement process; it operated independently of the Department of Health and Social Security and the Welsh Office, although it was funded by the Department of Health, who also agreed its work programme (Department of Health and Social Security/Welsh Office 1971).

The observational methods used neither national nor local standards. One of the observational studies was specific to mental health services for older people; neither was part of an enforcement process.

Development of methodologies

The questionnaire survey

Because the literature relating to the development of methodologies for evaluating health and social care was not consistent in all the topics covered, where feasible, key people involved in each of the evaluation programmes were contacted, and asked to complete a questionnaire, to provide information about aspects of the development of the methodology.

The organisations or people contacted were: the JCAHO, USA; the CCHSA, Canada; the ACHS, Australia; KFOA/HQS and the HAP, UK; Standards for Australian Nursing Homes; the WHO; the SSI, UK, in relation to both their inspections, and 'best value'; joint reviews; the Audit Commission, in relation to 'best value'; and one of the authors regarding the observational method.

Those contacted were asked whether, in the development of standards, and of other aspects of the programme, an evidence base (for example, literature review), and consultation with professionals, service users and carers were used.

The findings, based on the information provided by those organisations that replied, are summarised in Table 22.2. All the programmes contacted used an evidence base in developing standards. The evidence used included literature, guidance, standards used by similar schemes elsewhere, and original research. Half the schemes applied an evidence base in developing other aspects of the programmes, using the same sources as for the standards.

Table 22.2: Features in the development of the methodology of approaches to evaluating health and social care

	CCHSA	KFOA/ HQS	HAP	SSI	BV (SSI)	Obs
Evidence-based standards	✓	✓	✓	✓	✓	✓
Evidence-based other	✓	✓	✓	(✓)	(✓)	×
Consultation with professionals re: standards	✓	✓	✓	✓	✓	(✓)
Consultation with professionals re: other	✓	✓	✓	✓	✓	×
Consultation with users re: standards	×	✓	✓	✓	✓	×
Consultation with users re: other	×	×	✓	✓	✓	×
Consultation with carers re: standards	×	(✓)	x	✓	✓	×
Consultation with carers re: other	(✓)	(✓)	x	✓	✓	×

CCHSA: Canadian Council on Health Services Accreditation
KFOA/HQS: King's Fund Organisational Audit/Health Quality Service
HAP: Hospital Accreditation Programme
SSI: Social Services Inspectorate
BV: Best value (SSI)
Obs: Observational method (Clark and Bowling 1989)

All schemes except the observational study consulted professional organisations and individuals in developing both the standards, and other aspects of the programme.

Four of the six schemes contacted consulted users in the development of standards. The CCHSA consulted surveyors and professionals, but the question was more specifically about users of services. Only half the schemes consulted users in developing other aspects of the programme.

Carers were the least consulted group. Only two of the six schemes (both run by the SSI) contacted included them specifically, in developing the standards and other aspects of the programme.

Of the schemes contacted in this exercise, those with the soundest base, in terms of evidence and consultation, were those run by the SSI, which, for both its normal inspections, and 'best value', answered 'yes' to all the above questions; the partial exception was an evidence base for aspects of the approach other than standards, for which they said they held a briefing for inspection teams. Presumably, this indicated that the teams were consulted about the approach to be used, whereas, ideally, wider consultation before this event would be desired. The next most sound basis was that of the HAP, which answered' yes' to all the questions, except those relating to carers. They felt that organisational standards, on the whole, had less relevance for carers than clinical standards.

The observational method carried out no consultation on the approach to be used, although, as may be expected in a research study of this kind, the measures used were based on evidence.

Other programmes

In addition to the information obtained through the postal exercise described above, features of other evaluation programmes, relating to the topics covered in the postal exercise, are as follows.

The EFQM improved model was tested and reviewed by more than 500 model users in Europe, prior to presentation in 1999 at the EFQM representatives meeting in Geneva, where it was accepted.

In devising standards for residential and nursing homes for older people, for the NCSC, the CPA established an advisory group, encompassing all the key interests in the field, held meetings with providers, regulators and services users, visited homes and reviewed research. The Department of Health then consulted on the draft standards before publication (Department of Health 2001a).

The SSI publication *Inspecting for Quality: standards for the residential care of elderly people with mental disorders* (Department of Health, Social Services Inspectorate 1993) was produced by a small group of Inspectorate and Department of Health staff, after consultation with representatives of users and providers in the field.

The standards contained in the *Alzheimer's Disease Society Quality Assurance Initiative* (Alzheimer's Disease Society 1996) were consulted on with carers, people with dementia, volunteers and staff.

The CHI's evidence framework for the first clinical governance reviews in health authorities and primary care was consulted on with a range of statutory and voluntary agencies and organisations representing service users, carers and people from ethnic minorities, and a similar consultation exercise was carried out in relation to the evidence framework for the first clinical governance reviews of mental health services.

The JCAHO in 1982 added public members to its governing board, and in 1999 formed a Public Advisory Group on Healthcare Quality, to advise the board on policy issues, in response to pressure from the public.

These findings reinforce those from the organisations contacted in the postal exercise, that professionals in the field and service users are relatively well consulted in the development of standards and approaches for evaluating health and social care. Voluntary organisations are sometimes perceived as having a more radical, user-focused approach than others; it is perhaps not surprising, therefore, that the Alzheimer's Disease Society consulted with carers, people with dementia and volunteers.

The Health Advisory Service (HAS 2000) used an evidence base, from the relevant literature, in the development of standards, and in the development of other aspects of the programme, in that it based its approach on other similar schemes. It consulted with professional organisations, royal colleges, and organisations representing services users and carers in the development of standards and of other aspects of the programme, through the advisory groups and advisory networks which were established. For its mental health services for older people standards programme, focus groups of users and carers were also held, for additional work on standards development.

PART VIII

DEVELOPING STANDARDS TO EVALUATE MENTAL HEALTH SERVICES FOR OLDER PEOPLE

CHAPTER 23

The method used

Introduction

In this chapter, an account is given of the method devised by the Health Advisory Service (HAS 2000) to evaluate mental health services for older people. A similar process was used in developing the evaluation instruments and methodologies for all the client groups covered by HAS (the others were adult mental health, mentally disordered offenders, child and adolescent mental health services and care of older people). The account covers the structures created in order to develop the methodology, the development of the standards which formed the basis of the service evaluations, consultation on those standards, the pilot service reviews, and the mechanisms used to test the validity and reliability of the standards. The background to HAS 2000 is given in Chapter 21, and validity and reliability are also discussed in Chapters 25 to 27.

Advisory groups

A development team was established, comprising 10 senior people from a range of professions and interests, including old age psychiatry, nursing, clinical psychology, occupational therapy, public health, social work and the voluntary sector. They advised on the use of the results of content analysis, together with already-existing protocols, to draft the new evaluation instrument for mental health services for older people, considered comments received as a result of postal consultations (see below), and some members were reviewers on pilot service reviews (see below). An advisory network was created, consisting of 100 organisations and individuals with an interest in the field. Members were invited to take part in consultation on the standards, and the network membership was later pruned to 60, when those who did not respond to these invitations were removed from the list.

Selection of the literature

A literature search was undertaken of the main relevant publications relating to mental health services for older people over the previous 10 years, in order to draw up a list of the main documents in the field, for content analysis. A draft list was circulated for comment to key people (mainly consultant psychiatrists, and colleagues from some other disciplines, for example clinical psychologists), leading to the creation of a definitive list of 26 publications to be considered and categorised according to priority for content analysis.

Content analysis

In order that information could be extracted from the literature in a consistent way, to inform the development of standards, a method of content analysis was devised, which was based on the academic construct grounded theory. Unlike quantitative data analysis techniques, it does not impose an external structure on the data, but instead the systematic analysis of documents enables themes, patterns and categories to be teased out. The framework used was based on the work of Easterby-Smith *et al.* (1991), who describe seven main stages, as follows.

1 *Familiarisation*: the exploratory stage, in which data are examined and framing of questions is started.
2 *Reflection*: a process of evaluation and critique, as the data are evaluated in the light of previous research, texts and ideas.
3 *Conceptualisation*: the set of variables or concepts derived from the two previous stages are examined from the point of view of their reliability or validity.
4 *Cataloguing concepts*: decisions are made regarding the categorisation or 'labelling' of themes.
5 *Re-coding*: this stage involves returning to the data, testing the categories and re-coding for refinement.
6 *Linking*: data and categories are linked with more general models, considered in stage 2, and a more holistic theory begins to emerge.
7 *Re-evaluation*: in the light of the comments of others, first conceptualisations are re-written, taking into account criticisms made and contradictions highlighted. This stage may continue for a considerable period of time, and, as with other stages, it may have to be undertaken more than once.

Based on this framework, a system of content analysis was devised, within which statements from the relevant literature were categorised according to subject of statement, type of statement and client orientation. The subject of statement category comprised clinical and therapeutic practice, service provision, commissioning practice, and evaluation and development methods, the first three of which included further sub-classifications. Statements, once categorised, were indexed to indicate the type of statement: the types were legal requirement, government body directive, research-based statement, recommendations from documents based on advice, consensus and statements from organisations or individuals, examples of good practice, issues discussed in documents which affected purchasing or provision, and other. Statements were then indexed to show their client orientation, in terms of age group and specific client group.

Training was provided for all those who carried out the content analysis, which included practice in completing the content analysis pro-forma, discussion of issues arising in carrying out the process, and the timetable and procedures for completing the exercise. Fourteen content analyses were completed for this client group.

Service mapping

In order to create suitable section headings for the draft evaluation instrument, a 'mapping services' exercise was carried out. All aspects of commissioning and providing services for older people with mental health problems, by health and social services, were included on a 'map'. Discussion with the development team was important in ensuring that all topics were covered. So that sections of the instrument, and the standards within them, would relate to factors which contributed to really effective services for users, the user's experience of services at the various stages was used as a reference point.

Drafting the evaluation instrument

To create the first draft evaluation instrument, statements were taken from the completed content analyses and placed under the headings formed from the mapping services exercise. Statements referring to similar topics were then grouped together, and written as standards and criteria. Subsequent drafts were produced, incorporating changes indicated as a result of consultation and pilot service reviews (*see* Chapter 22).

Consultation

This section describes the methods used for consultation on the standards. These were postal consultations and a consultative conference, involving the advisory network, a postal consultation with professional organisations, and focus groups with users and carers. By obtaining assessments of the presentation and relevance of the standards, and addressing the issues of whether they appeared to be relevant, reasonable, unambiguous and clear, the consultative conference, the postal consultations with the advisory network and the postal consultation with professional organisations were means of testing their face validity (Bowling 1997).

Through addressing the extent to which the standards instrument appeared to logically examine and comprehensively include, in a balanced way, the full scope of the characteristic or domain it was intended to measure, the consultative conference, the postal consultations with the advisory network and the postal consultation with professional organisations, and the focus groups with users and carers were means of testing the standards' content validity (Bowling 1997). The types of validity are discussed further in Chapter 25.

Postal consultations

The first postal consultation took place when those members of the advisory network not able to attend the consultative conference were given the option of submitting their comments by post or telephone. Eleven members responded in this way. The second was carried out following the pilot evaluation visits (*see* Chapter 24), when a mailing was sent to the revised membership of the advisory network, inviting members to assist in editing the current draft of the evaluation instrument. Using a standards-only version (the criteria accompanying the standards were omitted), they were asked to rate each of the standards, to indicate their importance in the provision of good quality mental health services for older people, and 17 responses were received. They were also asked to edit a section of the document, comprising both standards and criteria, identifying what they perceived as duplications relating to standards or criteria in the sections, or gaps in section headings, standards or criteria. Twenty-two responses were received. The third postal consultation took place when, following the editing of all HAS 2000's evaluation instruments for all its client groups, for consistency, a final draft was sent to members of the advisory network, for their comments. They were invited to comment on the document, and in particular on whether, in re-organising the contents of the instrument, anything had been lost, and whether the standards and criteria had retained their meaning. Seven members responded. In addition, 47 professional organisations were sent drafts of the evaluation instruments for those client groups which it was considered they would be interested in, inviting their comments. Nine organisations submitted comments relating to mental health services for older people. In order to ensure consistency of approach, responses received from the postal consultations, and the proposed revisions to the evaluation instrument, were agreed at meetings of the development team.

Consultative conference

All members of the advisory network were invited to a conference, to discuss and comment on the draft standards, and 35 attended. The purpose of the conference was to reach consensus on standards and criteria in the draft evaluation instrument. The objectives of the conference were to:

- develop an instrument that has general acceptability and validity across a range of groups
- carry out meaningful consultation on the draft standards, with the range of parties concerned ('meaningful' here meant consultation that would be effective, and lead to actual changes to the draft standards)
- achieve better quality in the discussion about, and subsequent refinement of, the draft standards, than would be possible by post and telephone only
- publicise the evaluation framework
- gain acceptance of the standards, and the framework, in the field.

Participants were divided into workshops, to work on linked sections of the draft evaluation instrument. Members of the workshops were given the remit to edit and revise the standards and criteria, producing 3–5 standards and 10–15 criteria for each defined area. Areas could be amalgamated, or new ones created if necessary.

Four of the six workshops were chaired by members of the development team, and this was found to be particularly beneficial, since, having been closely involved with the development of the evaluation instrument, they had a good grasp of the background to the conference and the issues involved, and were familiar with the instrument.

Focus groups

The author held focus group meetings with users and carers (Finch and Orrell 1999) with the aim of ensuring that the content of the standards covered the issues that they considered most important. Meetings were held initially with two user groups and one carers' group. The user groups were for older people with functional mental illness, mainly depression, most of whom had previously attended a local day hospital. The carers' group, for those looking after older people with dementia, was held at the day centre that the person they cared for attended.

Five users were present in one group, and eight in the other, and eight carers were present at the carers' support group meeting. In addition to the group members, colleagues who normally facilitated the groups were involved in the exercise. These were senior occupational therapists, a deputy ward manager, and a day services officer.

A written document was created, comprising questions based on the draft standards. The main themes and topics addressed in the standards were summarised, and re-worded with the aim of rendering them jargon-free and user-friendly. Headings were created, and questions for discussion were included beneath each heading. The written questions were sent to the group facilitators prior to the focus group meetings. In the case of the two user groups, the facilitators started to discuss these with group members before the planned sessions. The author attended a meeting of the carers' group, and gave a brief talk about the standards, before arranging the more focused session.

The group discussions were flexibly structured around the questions. The discussions were either led by the author, with input from the normal facilitator, or vice versa. Each group concentrated on one main heading in the questions document, such as 'The kinds of services provided', or 'Making sure that people get the services they need'. In one of the user groups, the exercise continued during normal group meetings after the planned focus group session, and all the headings in the questions document were covered. The author and the group facilitators then met, and the group's responses to all the questions were drawn together.

Because this exercise proved to be so informative, it was repeated. For the second round of focus groups, the author again met two groups of older people with functional mental illness, and one group of carers of older people with dementia. Three members were present at one of the user groups, and two at the other, and 10 members were present at the carers' group. As before, the workers who normally facilitated the groups attended. These were a psychotherapist, an occupational therapy technician and an outreach worker. The method used was the same as for the first round of meetings. For the second round of meetings, the author facilitated all the group discussions, and the normal group facilitator joined in the discussion, clarifying any points as appropriate.

The main issues that arose from the focus groups were as follows.

- If group members, or someone close to them, had mental health problems, they would normally turn to their general practitioner (GP) for help initially. However, it was reported that some GPs did not have the necessary depth of knowledge about mental health, or did not have sufficient time to spend talking to users about their problems.
- Provision of transport was seen as crucial for some users to attend services, for example day hospitals. Effective organisation of transport was also thought to be important. It was felt that it should arrive at the user's home at the time agreed, that it should be warm and comfortable, and that the length of journey time for each user should be reasonable.
- Consistency for users in the input of the various disciplines concerned was thought to be required. It was reported that junior doctors, occupational therapists and psychologists rotated, and that since users are in contact with services for older people longer than is the case with acute care, the changes in personnel were noticed more. It was remarked that some consultants were never seen, and that instead, a patient may see a series of registrars, who cover for a consultant.
- In inpatient services, there was a perceived need for better communication with users about their care. It was felt that they should be welcomed to the ward, and that someone should explain to them, what would happen during their stay. Similarly, it was thought that more consideration should be given to communication with relatives and carers. An example was given of a user being given medication at different times than when at home, and of this not being discussed with the carer, who was concerned.
- In relation to complaints, it was suggested that it should be possible to make these confidentially. Group members feared that those responsible would 'take it out on you' if you complained.
- From the carers' point of view, it was thought important to have the facility for a care worker to be based in the home when required, including at night-times.
- It was felt that sufficient day care should be provided, so that users who wished to attend could do so.

A new standard and nine new criteria were added to the standards document for mental health services for older people as a result of the views gathered from the groups.

Editing the standards

Following consultation and piloting (*see* Chapter 24), the evaluation instrument, together with those for all HAS 2000's client groups, was edited, with the aim of achieving consistency between the instruments, prior to publication.

The levels system

The standards for each client group were re-arranged, using a system of levels, based on a model designed by the Royal College of Psychiatrists' Research Unit (Royal College of Psychiatrists' Research Unit 1996, unpublished). The levels were based on the concepts of the main 'customer' and the main 'actor'. The customer was the direct recipient of the action, and the actor was the person responsible for doing the action. The levels are shown in Table 23.1.

Table 23.1: Levels system for editing standards (based on Royal College of Psychiatrists' Research Unit, 1996, unpublished)

Level	Customer	Actor
1: Service delivery	User/carer	Front-line clinical or social care worker
2: Organisation of care	User/carer	Manager (may be clinician working in management capacity, e.g. ward manager)
3: Intra-agency organisational issues	Member of staff	Usually senior manager
4: Planning, integration and commissioning	The organisation	Service planners, senior managers, commissioners; those working at strategic level

The editing process

The standards and criteria in the draft evaluation instruments were mapped against the levels described above. This showed to what extent subject areas in the levels above were covered in the instruments, and gave an indication of which headings should be retained. Second order headings were devised, based on the pattern of standards and criteria that emerged. The text of the standards and criteria in the draft instruments was then re-ordered, into the levels, and the second order headings within them. Where it was appropriate for standards or criteria to be made the same across client groups, this was done. Common introductory and background sections were created, and a common referencing system was used.

CHAPTER 24

Pilot evaluations and reviews of services

Pilots

The sites

Two NHS trusts offered to be pilot sites for HAS 2000 reviews of mental health services for older people, and the pilots were undertaken in 1998. Both of the trusts' catchment areas included urban and rural parts. In the first site, the catchment area had a total population of approximately 290 000, and a population of those aged over 65 of approximately 45 000. The trust's mental health services for older people comprised five inpatient wards (one admission and assessment; one respite care and assessment (dementia); one slow rehabilitation, respite care and continuing care; one continuing care (functional); and one continuing care (functional and frail)), four day care facilities (two day hospitals, a rural day care project; and a group held twice weekly at a community centre, for people with functional illnesses), and nine community resource teams, which were multidisciplinary in membership, and in most cases were jointly funded with social services. A memory clinic was held at the district general hospital, and three outpatient clinics were held, one at the district general hospital weekly, and two at other locations in the area monthly. In addition, the service included psychology, occupational therapy, and arts therapies.

In the second site, the trust had a catchment area of approximately 200 000 people, and a population of those aged over 65 of approximately 35 000. The trust's mental health services for older people comprised two continuing care wards, a 'sub-acute' ward, an assessment ward, two day hospitals and a community mental health team. There were two geriatric rehabilitation wards at the district general hospital. The service also provided an outpatient service, and involvement with a memory disorders clinic, which was joint with the geriatric service.

The model used

The way in which the pilot evaluation visits were planned and carried out was broadly based on the model for visits to services adopted for use with the Clinical

Standards Advisory Group schizophrenia protocol (Wing *et al.* 1995). The service development adviser (SDA) (the author) managed the pilots, with support from HAS 2000 from a joint chief executive and the reviews administrator. For each pilot, an external review team of four people was used, with a specialist adviser acting as lead reviewer.

Method

A preliminary visit was made to the site by the SDA and the joint chief executive, at which key people were seen from the trust, the health authority, social services, and the voluntary sector, and main issues were highlighted. Information gathered was used in creating a profile of the service. This visit was also an opportunity for the SDA to become familiar with the district, and some of the places to be visited during the pilot. Documents such as strategies, procedures and service descriptions were requested from agencies at the site prior to the visit, and the SDA drew on these to prepare a briefing pack for review team members.

A key person at the review site was identified early in the process, as the main contact for the SDA and the reviews administrator. This person was a project manager in one case, and the personal assistant to the general manager of the Mental Health Directorate, in the other. The SDA provided this person with details of categories of people and places to be seen during the review. The key contact person then arranged the timetable for both the preliminary visit, and the review visit.

The pilot reviews each lasted three days, with a review team briefing meeting at the hotel on the evening immediately beforehand. The review team members included a consultant psychiatrist, a professor of clinical psychology of the elderly, an elderly services manager, the manager of a day hospital, a carer, and the SDA. Some members of the development team took part in the review teams for the pilots. This was helpful, both because they were familiar with the draft instrument, and because the group cohesion that had developed, aided collaborative working in the review team.

During the reviews, meetings were held with chief and senior officers at the NHS trusts, the (then) health authorities and social services, and clinicians and other staff from the trusts and social services, users and carers. Visits were made to wards, day hospitals, community teams, physiotherapy and arts therapy departments, nursing and residential homes, and voluntary organisations.

During the reviews, the four review team members divided into two pairs, to carry out these meetings and visits, so that more could be held than would otherwise have been the case. For each visit or meeting, the relevant standards and criteria from the draft evaluation instrument were considered. Each team member took on responsibility for a number of sections of the draft evaluation instrument. Although each member could not attend every meeting at which issues relevant to all those sections would be discussed, they would ask other team members to collect the information, and ensure that this was passed to them during the review. Team members completed the evaluation instrument by rating criteria as met, part met or not met, with comments to support the rating.

Review team meetings

A review team briefing meeting was held on the evening immediately prior to the review, to clarify the purpose of the review, go through the timetable in detail, decide which team members would attend which visits and meetings, examine the draft evaluation instrument, and explain practical details.

Each evening during the pilot, a meeting of the review team was held, to consolidate the day's findings, identify standards and criteria in the instrument for which information still needed to be gathered, decide which standards should be addressed during each of the visits and meetings to take place the following day, and make any necessary amendments to the allocation of review team members to those visits and meetings.

On the final afternoon of the pilot, a meeting was held to consolidate the information collected during the pilot, and start the process of drafting the final report. The aims of the meeting were to ensure that team members had all the information required in order to complete ratings and comments for the sections of the draft evaluation instrument for which they were responsible, to highlight the main issues that had emerged during the review, and to draft commendations and recommendations.

The review report

After the pilot review, the SDA prepared a draft report, based on team members' completed evaluation instruments, which was sent to team members for their comments. The revised draft was then sent to the site, for comment on factual accuracy, before being finalised. The review report comprised an introduction, background information about the service which was reviewed, an account of methods used during the review, detailed findings, commendations and recommendations.

Learning from the pilots

Some of the key points taken on board from the pilots were as follows.

- Familiarity with the evaluation instrument is crucial during review meetings and visits, review members have multiple tasks to undertake, and it is therefore important that they know their way around the instrument, in order to gather evidence effectively, in preparation for completing ratings.
- Where new reviewers are being used, it is beneficial to pair them up with more experienced reviewers, who are familiar with the process, and how to conduct the visits and meetings which make up a review.
- Suitable ways need to be found for review team members to talk with users and carers. Private space is required, so that users and carers can talk freely, and the location and time need to be convenient for them.

- If no user or carer groups exist, which may well be the case, special arrangements will need to be made. On the second pilot, review team members met carers in a private room at a day hospital which their relative attended, and this worked well.

Service reviews

Following the development of the evaluation instrument, including the piloting of the instrument and the review methods, as described above, the HAS started a programme of reviews of mental health services for older people, using the standards instrument. The methods used in the reviews were similar to those in the pilots, and were revised in the light of learning from those pilots. The review team comprised four or five people, managed by the SDA, and a week was spent at the site. The specialist adviser joined the team at the end of the week, to advise them in drawing conclusions from their findings. Following the production of the review report, the SDA and the specialist adviser, or another member of the review team, attended a meeting with key people from the service and their stakeholders, to present the report and discuss how the service planned to implement improvements.

PART IX

VALIDITY

CHAPTER 25

Achieving validity in standards

Introduction

In this section an account is given of the methods used to ensure that the Health Advisory Service (HAS) standards for mental health services for older people had validity. The background to validity is provided.

Validity is an assessment of whether an instrument measures what it aims to measure. An instrument is assigned validity after it has been satisfactorily tested repeatedly in the populations for which it was designed. This type of validity is known as internal validity, as opposed to external validity, which refers to the generalisability of the research findings to the wider population of interest (Bowling 1997). This study sought to determine the validity of the standards for mental health services for older people, both by a robust qualitative process of development, and by establishing the validity of the standards in practice.

Face validity

Face validity is often confused with content validity, but it is more superficial. It simply refers to investigators' subjective assessments of the presentation and relevance of, for example, a questionnaire: do the questions appear to be relevant, reasonable, unambiguous and clear? (Bowling 1997). For this study, a consultative conference, postal consultations with an advisory network and with professional organisations, and pilot evaluations of services (*see* Chapters 23 and 24) tested, and made further contributions to, the face validity of the HAS 2000 standards document (Health Advisory Service 2000 1999).

At the consultative conference, participants thought that many of the standards and criteria in the draft document were broadly of the right kind. However, a significant number were re-written. Some were found to address only part of a topic, for example gender alone, when it was considered appropriate to include minority ethnic issues also. Others were re-worded to reflect more accurately what participants felt to be priorities, for example by adding the word *real* to 'access to services', since access was perceived to be available sometimes in theory only. In a few instances, the status of criteria was changed, so that they became standards.

In the first postal consultation, there were proposals that the contents of the document should be re-organised, for example to make it more user-friendly, or more consistent. In the second postal consultation, the prioritisation exercise assisted in the process of reducing the number of standards and criteria, and comments made in the editing exercise contributed to changes in wording, for greater clarity, as did comments made in the consultation with professional organisations. In the pilot service evaluations, changes in the instrument were indicated, to achieve clarity in those sections of the document relating to continuing care, and to make it clear that all continuing care beds purchased by the NHS were included in reviews.

Content validity

This refers to judgements (usually made by a panel) about the extent to which the content of the instrument appears logically to examine and comprehensively include, in a balanced way, the full scope of the characteristic or domain it is intended to measure. The higher the content validity of a measure, the broader are the inferences that we can validly draw about a subject under a variety of conditions and in different situations. For this study, as in the case of face validity, a consultative conference, postal consultations with an advisory network and with professional organisations, and pilot evaluations of services (*see* Chapters 23 and 24) tested, and made further contributions to, the content validity of the HAS 2000 standards document (Health Advisory Service 2000, 1999).

The standard and criteria which were added to the instrument as a result of the focus groups (*see* Chapter 23), introduced topics, or aspects of topics, not identified by other means, and this also constituted a significant contribution to its content validity.

At the consultative conference, most section headings in the draft evaluation tool were found to be relevant. However, some changes were suggested for the commissioning section of the evaluation instrument, in particular to make it more 'future-proof', in the light of the Government White Paper *The New NHS: modern – dependable* (Secretary of State for Health 1997).

Because content analysis had been used to identify statements for use in the draft instrument, some sections had many more criteria than others. This was illustrated in particular in the case of the continuing care sections, which included long lists of criteria. Conference participants' views reinforced the point that this created an imbalance, and the document was revised accordingly.

In the first postal consultation, there were requests that particular disciplines be more adequately represented at appropriate points in the document. In the pilot service evaluations, changes in the instrument were indicated, to include how health and social services monitor continuing care, within both the NHS and the independent sector.

In addition to the mechanisms described above, an exercise was carried out, comparing the HAS 2000 standards with another document. As is shown elsewhere in this book (*see* Chapters 22 and 28), there is no other instrument to evaluate mental health services for older people which covers all aspects of the service. There was, therefore, no existing comparable instrument that could be used to test the validity of the HAS 2000 standards. An exercise was undertaken to create an instrument that could be used as a comparable indicator of what should be covered in services. The 'raw material' chosen for this was the World Health Organization (WHO) and World Psychiatric Association (WPA) (1998) consensus statement: *Organization of Care in Psychiatry of the Elderly – a technical consensus statement*. An aim of that document was to describe the basic components of care to older people with mental disorders, and their co-ordination. Subsequent stages of the exercise compared the HAS standards with the WHO and WPA statement.

The exercise used content analysis, following the method described in Chapter 23, that is to say, it was identical to the content analysis used to create statements for the draft HAS standards. The people who carried out the exercise for the WHO and WPA and HAS 2000 standards content analysis had received training for, and carried out, content analysis, in the earlier operation also.

The work was carried out in three stages, as follows.

Stage 1

Content analysis of the WHO and WPA article was completed, using the methodology described in Chapter 23.

Stage 2

Using the information extracted from the WHO and WPA article in the content analysis, statements were created that could be tested against the HAS 2000 standards. There were 30 such statements, and a table was devised, showing these.

Stage 3

In the table (Table 25.1), against the statements from the WHO and WPA article, were inserted the reference numbers of those standards from the HAS 2000 standards document which covered the content of each statement. The extent to which the WHO and WPA statements were covered by the HAS 2000 standards was assessed.

For 28 of the 30 statements produced from the content analysis of the WHO and WPA article, there were one or more standards from the HAS 2000 standards document which covered the statement. For two of the statements from the WHO and WPA article, there were no standards from the HAS 2000 standards document which covered the statement. There was thus 93% concordance between the WHO and WPA article and the HAS 2000 standards.

Table 25.1: Results of exercise to test content validity, using World Health Organization and World Psychiatric Association consensus statement and HAS 2000 standards

Content analysis of WHO/WPA consensus statement	HAS 2000 standards for MHSFOP
Statement (text)	Standards which cover content of statement (by level and number)
Early identification of mental health problems facilitates access to services.	
Preventive strategies for patients, families and carers should form an integral part of the service. These strategies need co-ordinating between all disciplines and with primary care and may include educational activities.	LIV:2.1
Initial assessment should be carried out at home where possible and may involve carers and families who may be in the best position to report a change in behaviour that may signify mental illness.	LI:1.1
Primary care teams are responsible for the initial identification and referral of patients.	LI:1.2
All care professionals should be trained in comprehensive initial assessment, the use of screening instruments as appropriate and good record keeping.	LI:1.1/LIII:6.2
Care of the elderly requires a strong contribution from Old Age Psychiatry.	
Services should be aiming to meet need within an appropriate cultural setting and in accordance with scientific knowledge and ethical requirements.	LII:2.1/LII:4.4/LIV:6.2
Patients, their families and carers have the right to participate in the planning of healthcare services.	LI:2.5/LII:8.2/ LIII:1.1/LIV:2.1/ LIV:6.2
Good quality of care for older people with mental health problems is comprehensive, accessible, responsive, individualised, trans-disciplinary, accountable, systematic.	LII:1.1/LII:4.2/LII:4.3
A diagnostic formulation is important not only to allow rational care planning but also to inform patients and carers of the situation, management options and prognosis.	LI:2.4/LII:4.4
Progress must be monitored in follow up and risk of relapse considered.	LI:2.6
The primary goal of management should be maintaining or improving the quality of life of patients and carers.	LI:2.1/LI:3.1
A proactive rather than crisis-driven service is more humane and efficient.	LI:2.6
A systematic multidisciplinary approach to record keeping and information sharing is highly desirable.	LII:4.4/LIII:7.4
Provision of flexible respite may be crucial for enabling informal carers to continue their role. Respite can be provided in or out of the home.	LI:2.4/LII:2.4/LII:6.1
Legal rights of patients in financial and other personal areas should be protected and may involve advocates and advance directives.	LII:2.3/LIII:1.6

Table 25.1: *Continued*

Content analysis of WHO/WPA consensus statement	HAS 2000 standards for MHSFOP
Statement (text)	*Standards which cover content of statement (by level and number)*
Although care should be provided in the patient's home as long as possible sometimes residential care is the only way of meeting the patient's needs.	LII:2.1/LIV:5.1
Spiritual and leisure needs should not be neglected.	LII:4.5/LIII:6.2
The community mental health team may consist of doctors, psychiatric nurses, psychologists, social workers, therapists and secretaries.	LII:2.1/LII:4.2/LIII:3.2
Provision of good service requires smooth transition from one service component to another.	LIII:2.1/LIV:5.1/ LIV:7.1
Community mental health teams are responsible for specialist assessment of older people at home.	LI:1.1
Inpatient units should provide assessment and treatment for the full range of mental disorders and rehabilitation.	LII:4.1/LII:7.1/LII:7.2
Day hospitals offer multidisciplinary assessment, diagnosis and treatment of patients that can be maintained at home.	LII:3.3
Outpatient services provide assessment, diagnosis and treatment of patients fit enough to attend; transport should be provided.	LII:1.1
Hospital respite should be available for patients with difficult behavioural problems associated with mental illness; these patients may also require continuing hospital care.	LII:6.1/LIV:2.2
Provisions for dying patients and their families should be made.	LI:2.2
Liaison services should be provided across the range of facilities for the elderly.	LII:7.1/LIV:7.1/ LIV:7.3
Formal and informal community support agencies enable the elderly to remain at home and may include home care, day care and self-help groups.	LI:2.4/LII:2.4
Good services are underpinned by good research, evaluation and training.	LII:7.1/LIII:3.1/ LIII:4.2/LIII:7.2/ LIV:9.1/LIV:9.2
Responsive action should lead to the development, appropriate to local conditions, of the components of service that will adequately address the needs of older people with mental health disorders.	LII:2.1/LII3.2/LII:5.1/ LIII:6.1/LIII:8.1/ LIV:1.1/LIV:2.2/ LIV:3.1

WHO/WPA: World Health Organization and World Psychiatric Association
MHSFOP: Mental Health Services for Older People
LI: Level I
LII: Level II
LIII: Level III
LIV: Level IV
The levels LI, LII, LIII or LIV refer to the levels system used in the HAS 2000 Standards for Mental Health Services for Older People (1999), and are inserted before the actual number of the standard to indicate the level in which each standard appears. For the purposes of this exercise, each standard referred to comprises both the standard itself, and its accompanying criteria.

PART X

TESTING THE RELIABILITY OF STANDARDS IN USE

CHAPTER 26

Reliability

Background

Reliability concerns the extent to which an experiment, test, or any measuring procedure yields the same results on repeated trials. Because repeated measurements never exactly equal one another, unreliability is always present to at least a limited extent. However, while repeated measurements of the same phenomenon never precisely duplicate each other, they do tend to be consistent from measurement to measurement. The person with the highest blood pressure on a first reading, for example, will tend to be among those with the highest reading on a second examination given the next day. The same will be true among the entire group of patients whose blood pressure is being recorded; their readings will not be exactly the same from one measurement to another, but they will tend to be consistent. This tendency towards consistency found in repeated measurements of the same phenomenon is referred to as reliability. The more consistent the results given by repeated measurements, the higher the reliability of the measuring procedure; conversely the less consistent the results, the lower the reliability (Carmines and Zeller 1994).

Errors in measurement

Empirical measurements are affected by random error and nonrandom error. Random error is the term used to designate all of those chance factors that confound the measurement of any phenomenon. The amount of random error is inversely related to the degree of reliability of the measuring instrument. The effects of random error are totally unsystematic in character. A scale that is affected by random error will sometimes overweigh a particular object and on other occasions underweigh it. Classical test theory, which is described below, is a model for assessing random measurement error. Unlike random error, nonrandom error has a systematic biasing effect on measuring instruments. Thus, a scale that always registers the weight of an object two pounds below its actual weight is affected by nonrandom measurement error (Carmines and Zeller 1994).

Standard deviation

Standard deviation (SD) is based on the difference of values from the mean value (the spread of individual results round a mean value). It is the most common measure of dispersion (a summary of a spread of cases in a figure) (Bowling 1997).

Classical test theory

In classical test theory, the assumption is that an individual test score (X) is the sum of two components: the true score (T) and a measurement error (E). In terms of simple algebra, this is: $X = T + E$. The 'true' score, T, is a hypothetical, unobservable, or latent quantity. It is defined in terms of the average score that would be obtained if the measurement process could be repeated indefinitely. In statistics this average is known as an expected value. T can be estimated, by the observed (guessed) score, for example, and some idea of the precision of this estimate may be obtained from the variability of the errors (measured by their SD, for example). In classical test theory, the SD of the errors is usually referred to as the standard error of measurement, or as repeatability (Dunn 1997).

Bias and precision

Dunn (1998) used the example of a piece of string to demonstrate bias and precision. He described an exercise whereby he invited the reader to take a piece of string and to guess its length, repeating the act several times. The average of the guesses (their arithmetic mean) would be the reader's best estimate of the string's actual length. Measuring the string with a rule would give the 'true' length; the difference between this 'true' length and the average would be a measure of the bias in the guesses (measurements). A measure of the variability of the guesses would provide an estimate of the reader's precision as a measuring instrument. The higher the reader's precision was, the lower the variability of their guesses would be. Variability is most commonly described through the use of the measurement's SD, or the square of the SD – the variance. The fluctuations of the guesses about their mean value may be regarded as random measurement errors. The SD of the guesses themselves is also the SD of the measurement errors. The standard error of measurement is the square root of the variance of the individual errors.

Generalisability theory

Generalisability (G) theory is a statistical theory about the dependability of behavioural measurements. Whereas classical test theory can estimate separately only one source of error at a time, the strength of G theory is that multiple sources of error in a measurement can be estimated separately in a single analysis. G theory enables the decision maker to determine how many occasions, test forms and administrators are needed to obtain dependable scores (Shavelson and Webb 1991).

Number of facets

A one-facet universe is defined by one source of measurement error, that is, by a single facet. If the decision maker intends to generalise from one set of test items to a much larger set of test items, *items* is a facet of measurement; the item universe would be defined by all admissible test items. If the decision maker is willing to generalise from one set of test forms to a much larger set of test forms, *forms* is a facet; the universe would be defined by all admissible test forms. If the decision maker is willing to generalise from performance on one occasion to performance on a much larger set of occasions, *occasions* is a facet; the occasions universe would be defined by all admissible occasions (Shavelson and Webb 1991).

Social science measures are more complex, and therefore contain more than one facet. In an example of a behavioural observation, the two-facet universe would be observers and occasions. An observer would watch a person and count, rate or score their behaviour. The frequency count, score or rating given by a particular observer would be used as an indication of the average frequency count, score or rating that would have been obtained with many observers. The greater the inconsistencies among observers in their ratings of behaviour, the more hazardous the generalisation from one observer's rating of behaviour to the universe of interest. Where items constituted a facet of the achievement measurement described above, here *observers* is recognised as a facet.

Repeated observations of behaviour are made commonly in both research and applied settings, in recognition that behaviour may vary from one occasion to the next. To the extent that behaviour is inconsistent across occasions, generalisation from the sample of behaviour collected on one occasion, to the universe of behaviour across all occasions of interest is hazardous. *Observation occasions* is therefore a second facet (Shavelson and Webb 1991).

The complexity of social science measures cannot always be captured by two facets. Student performance may vary over items and occasions. Test performance might also vary according to the clarity of the administrator's instructions, or the tone the administrator sets for the test. *Administrators*, then, would constitute a third facet; generalising from performance under one administrator to the average over all possible administrators may lead to error. The universe of admissible observations would then be defined by three facets – *items, occasions and administrators* – taken together (Shavelson and Webb 1991).

Designs for reliability studies

The design of a reliability study is dependent on the context within which the study is being undertaken, what sort of measuring instruments are being used or compared, and what properties or characteristics are being measured. There appear to be three main roles for reliability studies. These are:

- as an aid to instrument development (including training of interviewers, raters or examiners)

- as an aid to the choice of measuring instrument or to the choice of conditions under which measurements are to be made
- as a way of monitoring instrument use (quality control) (Dunn 1989).

Choice of subjects

When considering a measuring instrument, and assessing its potential usefulness, attention should be paid to the population of subjects on which it is to be used. For example, a test of cognitive ability might be useful in discriminating between the talents of individuals in a general population of school children, but be practically useless when used to monitor subtle changes in the abilities of a population of children with learning disability. The key question is 'Is the measuring instrument or technique capable of adequately fulfilling its intended role?'. In order to answer this question, an investigator is obliged to evaluate the method on subjects that are typical of those that will be encountered during its routine use (Dunn 1989).

Simple replications

The simplest design for a study of instrument precision involves repeated measurements on the same subjects using the same instrument under conditions that remain as stable as possible (Dunn 1989). If the measuring instruments are human raters (psychiatrists diagnosing different forms of madness in a group of psychotic patients, for example), then it is quite likely that the raters will remember their previous ratings or diagnoses and their assessments will be influenced by them. Usually they will give similar ratings or diagnoses in each of the replications. The results would suggest that raters' performance is better than it really is.

This effect of memory is not limited to the case where raters make subjective decisions. In a second attempt at a test of cognitive ability, a subject may remember his or her previous answers and simply repeat them. Someone filling in a questionnaire on political attitudes for the second time is also likely to remember the responses from the first time round and repeat them, to give a potentially misleading impression of stability. When measurements are made on living organisms, the characteristics being measured might change from one replication to another. In the behavioural and social sciences one needs to take measurements fairly closely together in time, so that there is little possibility of any underlying change. However, if they are too close, the subject, and the rater, may simply remember the previous response or rating, and repeat it (Dunn 1989).

Multiple indicators

Multiple indicators are used in situations where it is not possible to measure a characteristic at more then one time (Dunn 1989). In the behavioural and social sciences, many characteristics are not stable. One might, for example, wish to measure anxiety at a given point in an experiment, or immediately after presenting the subject with an aversive stimulus. In this situation, anxiety is a transient characteristic of a particular experimental condition (state anxiety as opposed to trait anxiety), and it needs to be assessed simultaneously through the use of two or more indicators. These indicators might be behavioural or physiological.

A further application of multiple indicators is in factor analytic models, used as a way of defining the concept being measured. It is impossible, for example, to obtain direct measurements of neuroticism, ambition, social status or racial prejudice. However, these concepts can be measured indirectly through the use of multiple indicator variables. Racial prejudice might be assessed from responses to several questions, such as, 'Do you have any friends who belong to a different ethnic background to your own?'.

Generalized staggered design

Generalized staggered design is one of many possible designs in the estimation of variance components for the two-way random model. In this design, half the raters for any one sample of subjects also rate the subjects for the neighbouring sample (Figure 26.1) (Dunn 1992). This was the design of the reliability study used to test the reliability of the HAS standards.

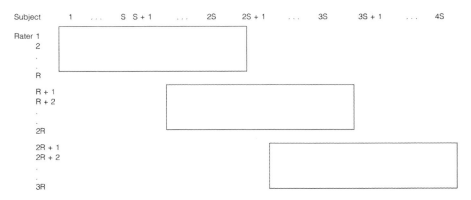

Figure 26.1: Generalized staggered design (Dunn 1992)
Dunn G (1992) Design and analysis of reliability studies. *Statistical Methods in Medical Research.* **1**: 123–57.

CHAPTER 27

Testing the reliability of the Health Advisory Service standards

Introduction

The aim was to ascertain the reliability of the standards, by measuring the variability of ratings, described through the standard deviation of the ratings. Since the raters to be used were in the main extremely busy people, a method to estimate reliability was required which involved a relatively small number of ratings to be carried out by each rater. Methods needing two testing situations were not, therefore, likely to be the most suitable. Since classical test theory would permit the estimation of only one source of error at a time, the application of G theory, was thought to be preferable. This would allow determination of how many occasions, test forms and administrators would be needed to obtain dependable scores. Generalised staggered design was considered suitable, partly because it is easy to carry out. In the actual design used for this study, each rater rated a minimum of 9 standards, and a maximum of 18, and most rated 16. The exercise could be seen as a decision (D) study, that is, making use of information gained to design the best possible application of the measurement for a particular purpose (Shavelson and Webb 1991). This study used a universe of generalisation of the facets: *standards, sites* and *raters*.

Instrument

As described in Chapter 24, the Health Advisory Service (HAS 2000) standards were designed to be used on systematic reviews of services, carried out by multiprofessional teams of assessors, who visit the site for several days. To arrange site visits of this nature to carry out an exercise to test the standards' reliability would not have been feasible, and it was, therefore, decided to undertake the test, using a written exercise. A 'standards-only' version of the standards document was produced, comprising standards, without the criteria which accompany them in the full standards document. Beneath each standard were included extracts from one or more of three reports of systematic reviews of mental health services for older people, which had been carried out at the three sites by multiprofessional teams, using the draft standards. The full standards document contained 75 standards. For this exercise, those standards for which there were no relevant statements in any of the three reports were excluded, leaving 59 standards. A check was carried out to ensure consistency of the text selected.

Raters

The raters used for the exercise were from the HAS advisory network for mental health services for older people (*see* Chapter 23). The network, of 60 people in total, consisted of senior professionals in this area of work, including practitioners and managers in the field, all of whom had previously taken part in consultation on the draft standards. They were thought to constitute ideal raters, since they were familiar with the issues, and were exactly the kind of people who would be reviewers on actual reviews.

Procedure

Following piloting of the process, for the reliability study all 60 people on the advisory network were invited to take part in the study, and 26 indicated that they were willing to do so. Both raters and standards were randomly ordered and labelled, and raters and standards were then allocated to groups, as shown in Table 27.1.

Raters were asked to indicate, on the basis of the extracts, whether, for each site, the standard would be met, part met, or not met, i.e. to provide a rating for each site for which an extract was provided. The codes used for entering the data are shown in Table 27.2.

Nineteen sets of completed ratings were eventually received and analysed.

Table 27.1: Allocation of raters and standards for reliability study, using generalised staggered design

Raters	Standards
1–6	1–10
4–9	11–18
7–12	19–26
10–15	27–34
13–18	35–42
16–21	43–50
19–24	51–59

Table 27.2: Codes for data entry for reliability study

Type of data	Code
Standards	1–59
Raters	1–24 (with 2 reserves, 25 and 26)
Reports	A, B, C
Rating of standards:	
Met	2
Part met	1
Not met	0
Certainty of rating*:	
Certain	1
Uncertain	0

*Raters were given the option of putting a ? after the rating, if they felt there was uncertainty.

Analysis

References to individual standards use both the number allocated to that standard for the reliability study and, in brackets, the number used in the original standards document (level I,II,III, or IV, and number).

The data collected from the reliability study were analysed by standard, showing, for each standard, the total SD of the scores for all the ratings in relation to all three review reports. They were also analysed by standard and report, showing, for each standard, the average of score and SD in relation to all the ratings for each of the three review reports, and an overall average of score and overall SD of score for each standard. In the analysis of ratings by standard and report, overall, the standards performed well with regard to the SD of ratings. For example, for 51 out of 137 ratings (37.2%), there was perfect agreement. This result was encouraging in terms of the reliability of the application of the standards.

Various approaches were explored, using the SD, to see which would reveal significant characteristics of the standards. With regard to standards with a relatively low SD, an approach that revealed significant features of standards, was to examine those standards that had a SD of 0 for the ratings for two or more reports.

As shown in Table 27.2, above, the scores given by the raters for each review report for which there was an extract of evidence, in relation to each standard, were coded for data entry as follows: 0 = not met; 1 = part met; 2 = met. In the tables below, the 'Average of score (overall)' refers to the average of score for that standard, for all the ratings given, for all 3 reports; the 'Range of average of score across reports' shows the range of the average of scores given, from the overall average of scores relating to each of the three reports.

There were 13 standards in this category; they are shown in Table 27.3, and are discussed below. Consideration was also given to relatively high SD. Only three standards (20 (III7.3), 30 (II8.1) and 44 (IV6.2)) had a SD above the overall SD (0.67) for one report. It was, therefore, decided to examine standards that had a SD above the overall SD for one report. These standards are included in Table 27.4, and are discussed below.

Rating of standards as met, part met or not met

The standards that had a SD of 0 for two or more reports had been mainly rated as unmet or part met (coded as 0 or 1). Of the 13 standards in this category, all the average of scores for the reports were below the overall average of score of 0.65, with a range of average of scores across the reports rated of 0–1, except for standard 15. The opposite was the case for the standards that had a SD above the average SD of 0.67 for one report: more had been rated as met (coded as 2). Of the three standards in this category, two had an average of scores for the reports above the overall average of score of 0.65, with a range of average of scores across the reports rated of 0.33–1.33, and one had an average of score for the reports below the overall average of score of 0.65, with a range of average of scores across the reports rated of 0–1.

Table 27.3: Standard deviation by standard and report, for standards with a standard deviation of 0 for two or more reports

Standard*	SD of score by report			Average of score (overall)	Range of average of score across reports
	A	B	C		
2 (III1.6)	0	0.58	0	0.50	0–1
7 (II2.3)	0	0		0	0
10 (II5.1)	0.50	0	0	0.08	0–0.25
12 (IV8.1)	0	0		0	0
14 (II2.4)	0	0.50	0	0.75	0.25–1
15 (IV9.2)	0.58	0	0	1.83	1.5–2
22 (III1.1)	0.50	0	0	0.42	0–1
24 (III8.1)	0.58	0	0	0.50	0–1
32 (IV6.3)	0.58	0	0	0.44	0–1
34 (IV2.1)	0.58	0	0	0.44	0-1
39 (IV9.1)	0	0		0	0
42 (II4.2)	0	0	0.55	0.80	0.4–1
48 (III2.1)	0	0	0.40	0.61	0-1

Table 27.4: Standard deviation by standard and report, for standards with a standard deviation above the overall standard deviation (0.67) for one report

Standard*	SD of score by report			Average of score (overall)	Range of average of score across reports
	A	B	C		
20 (III7.3)	0.82	0		0.50	0-1
30 (II8.1)	1.15	0.58	0.58	0.78	0.33–1.33
44 (IV6.2)	0.82			1.33	1.33

*Reference to standard in original standards document (level I,II,III, or IV, and number) is included in brackets.

Table 27.5: Overall average of score and overall standard deviation of score, by report

	Report			Overall
	A	B	C	
Overall average of score	0.72	0.69	0.51	0.65
Overall standard deviation of score	0.71	0.65	0.62	0.67

This would indicate that the rating of standards rated as unmet or part met (coded 0 or 1) was more reliable than that for those rated as met (coded as 2). This is likely to be because it is easier, on the basis of evidence provided, to see that a standard is not met, than that it is met. In order to see that it is met, several criteria would need to be fulfilled, and the evidence given may not cover all the criteria. This proposition is borne out by an examination of the overall average of score, and overall standard deviation of score, by report. As may be seen in Table 27.5, the overall average of score descends, in a sliding scale, from report A, through report B, to report C. The overall SD of score descends, following exactly the same pattern.

With regard to standard 15 (IV9.2), which had a SD of 0 for two or more reports, but, unlike the other standards in this category, had an average of scores for the reports that was above the overall average of score of 0.65, this may be explained by the nature of the extracts of evidence from the three review reports. For two reports, the extracts of evidence from the reports provided unequivocal evidence that the standard was met; for one report, however, the extract was more ambiguous.

The standard was:

Research in the mental health of older people is being carried out.

With regard to reports B and C, for which the SD was 0, the evidence was clear:

B: The standard, which relates to research in the mental health of older people, was fully met, using the existing criteria. The review team felt that, considering the proximity of the university, more use could be made of local opportunities for collaboration. The team was pleased to note that [the service] have a research group. In order to encourage participation in research, it is suggested that a programme of multidisciplinary training in research methods be established.

C: The review team noted that important research was being carried out in the trust, and at the ... centre, on the ... site, which was relevant to mental health and older people. The team could see scope for more links to be made between researchers, in order to maximise the benefits of findings.

With regard to report A, for which, unlike for reports B and C, the standard deviation was above 0, this may be because the extract of evidence was more ambiguous. It also introduced the topic of a programme of research, which was not specifically mentioned in the standard:

A: Dr ... [psychiatrist] had in 1993 been involved in an important multicentre study of maintenance of remission of depression with antidepressants and Dr ... [psychologist] is involved in innovative research (e.g. therapeutic groups, counselling and dementia care). However, there is no clear programme of research across the trust, partly as there is only one permanent psychiatrist. Assistant psychologists involved in doing research have been funded by the trust, with additional funding coming from R&D money.

Of the raters who rated standard 15, for report A, two rated it as met, and two as part met; for reports B and C, all rated it as met. None indicated that they were unsure about their ratings.

Standards that had a standard deviation (SD) above the overall SD for one report

Consideration is now given to those standards that had a SD above the overall SD of 0.67 for one report. In the case of standard 20 (III7.3), which had a SD above the overall SD of 0.67 for report A, this may be due to the nature of the extract of evidence used in the rating exercise. The standard would seem to be clear and unambiguous:

There is evidence of an audit cycle.

However, the evidence for report A may be open to different interpretations:

A: Audit in general would appear to be neither consistent nor planned across the various groupings, with the exception of the commendable audit work carried out in nursing (patient notes, care planning, report writing and developing an audit cycle).

Of the four raters who rated this standard, for report A, two rated the standard as part met, one as met, and one as not met. None indicated that they were unsure about their ratings.

The evidence for report B, however, for which the score had a SD of 0, would appear to be more categorical:

> B: ... there was no evidence of a consistent approach to audit, nor of implementation plans for changes in practice, in response to quality findings.

Of the four raters who rated this standard, for report B, all rated it as not met. None indicated that they were unsure about their ratings. (As report C did not include evidence for this standard, no extract of evidence was included for this report.)

In the cases of standards 30 (II8.1) and 44 (IV6.2), the SD may have been higher than the overall SD because too much material was packed into the standards statement. Standard 30 is considered first:

> Up-to-date and accurate information on a range of health and social care-related issues is readily available to users and carers, to cover all stages of the process of care.

This standard, in effect, comprises four parts, which are that information:

- is available to users and carers
- is up to date and accurate
- is on a range of health and social care-related issues
- covers all stages in the process of care.

With regard to the extracts of evidence for reports B and C, for which the SD was 0.58 in both cases, it was relatively clear that the standard was not fully met:

> B: For mental health problems, only verbal information was available. Written information about services was not always available and displayed in health settings, though other settings were not visited by the review team.

> C: with regard to information and support offered to [carers] in their role as a carer, practical support, such as respite and day care, were not always given. Carers are not routinely given copies of care plans.
>
> In terms of assessment in their own right, carers were not generally made aware of the Carers (Recognition and Services) Act 1995, and counselling was not available for all.

Of the raters who rated this standard, for report B, two rated it as part met, and one as unmet. For report C, two rated it as not met, and one as part met.

In relation to the extract of evidence for report A, however, for which the SD was 1.15, although the statement was clear:

'there appeared to be extensive information available for users and carers'

this statement actually only provided evidence for one part of the standard, that is, part 1), as described above. It gave no evidence for the other parts of the standard, parts 2), 3), and 4).

Of the raters who rated this standard, for report A, two rated it as met, and one as not met. None of the raters who rated standard 20 indicated that they were unsure about any of their ratings.

With regard to standard 44:

Commissioners have consulted with key partners to produce the population needs assessment and strategy for mental health services for older people, and to plan services.

This standard actually comprises three parts, which are that commissioners have consulted with key partners to:

• produce the population needs assessment for mental health services for older people
• produce the strategy for mental health services for older people
• plan services.

Only report A contained evidence that related to this standard, and the SD of the score was 0.82. The extract was:

The health authority has consulted with a wide range of people including [a voluntary organisation] on the production of the strategy document.

This extract only provided evidence in relation to part 2) of the standard, as described above. It gave no evidence for parts 1) or 3).

Of the raters who rated standard 44, for report A, three rated it as met, two as part met, and one as not met. None of the raters who rated standard 44 indicated that they were unsure about any of their ratings.

Differences between reports

The examples discussed above demonstrate that, in relation to standards 15 (IV9.2), 20 (III7.3), 30 (II8.1) and 44(IV6.2) the evidence from report A was ambiguous, or open to different interpretations, compared with that from reports B and C, or only provided evidence for one part of the standard. Consideration is given here to factors contributing to this. Firstly, the procedure used for providing overall ratings for each standard on reviews is discussed. For reports B and C, a pro-forma was utilised, comprising all the standards and their accompanying criteria, and space for ratings for all of these. The documented evidence collected from the review team was used to complete in the pro-forma individual ratings of met, part met or not met for each criterion accompanying each standard, wherever the review had produced evidence in relation to that criterion, and an overall rating was then given for each standard. The evidence provided in the text of the final review report, and therefore in the extracts of evidence in the rating exercise carried out for this study, were based on that rating exercise. For report A, this procedure was not followed, although the standards and criteria were used on the review.

A further difference between report A and reports B and C, and which in fact contributed to the difference in approach described above, was that the service development adviser (SDA) who managed the review, and wrote the final report, for report A was different from the SDA who managed the reviews and wrote the final reports for reports B and C.

Performance of standards by level

As described in Chapter 23, within the standards document, the standards were categorised into four levels, as follows: Level I: Service Delivery; Level II: Organisation of Care; Level III: Intra-Agency Organisational Issues; Level IV: Planning, Integration and Commissioning. The reliability of the standards' performance in relation to the levels used in the standards document was considered, using analysis by standard. Table 27.6 shows the standards in their levels, with their SD, and the number of standards in each level with a SD below and above the overall SD of 0.67, with percentages in brackets.

As may be seen from Table 27.6, the standards in every level performed well in terms of their SD. The proportion of standards with a SD below the overall SD was between 70% and 100%. In terms of consideration by standard and report, it was shown earlier in this chapter that looking at standards that had a SD of 0 for two or more reports, or a SD above the overall SD of 0.67 for one report, was a useful way of identifying significant features of standards. Using this approach, there were no standards that had a SD of 0 for two or more reports, or a SD above the overall SD of 0.67 for one report, in level I. In both level II and level III, there were four standards with a SD of 0 for two or more reports, and one standard with a SD above the overall SD of 0.67 for one report. In level IV there were five standards with a SD of 0 for two or more reports, and one standard with a SD above the overall SD of 0.67 for one report. None of the levels contained more than one standard with a SD above the overall SD of 0.67. Looking at standards that had a SD of 0 for two or more reports, which indicates good performance in relation to the SD, it may be seen that the rating of standards in level I was less reliable than that in the other levels. The level with the greatest number of standards with a SD of 0 for two or more reports was level IV. Standard 15(IV9.2) was from this level, and was the only standard that had a SD of 0 for two or more reports, for which the average score of the reports (1.83) was above the overall average of score of 0.65.

Table 27.6: Standards by level, with standard deviation

Level	Standards	SD<0.67	SD>0.67
I	3 (I 2.4), SD 0.45/ 4 (I 2.3), SD 0.49/ 27 (I 1.2), SD 0.52/ 43 (I 1.1), SD 0.39/ 50 (I 1.3), SD 0.52/ 51 (I 2.1), SD 0.46/ 58 (I 2.6), SD 0.52/ 59 (I 2.2), SD 0.41	8 (100)	0 (0)
II	5 (II 8.2), SD 0/ 7 (II 2.3), SD 0/ 8 (II 7.1), SD 0.72/ 10 (II 5.1), SD 0.29/ 14 (II 2.4), SD 0.45/ 17 (II 4.1), SD 0.79/ 19 (II 1.1), SD 0.45/ 23 (II 5.3), SD 0.35/ 26 (II 6.1), SD 0.78/ 30 (II 8.1), SD 0.83/ 35 (II 2.1), SD 0.52/ 36 (II 2.2), SD 0.52/ 38 (II 3.1), SD 0.42/ 41 (II 4.5), SD 0.82/ 42 (II 4.2), SD 0.41/ 46 (II 4.3), SD 0.41/ 54 (II 3.3), SD 0.51/ 55 (II 5.2), SD 0.39/ 56 (II 3.2), SD 0.55/57 (II 7.2), SD 0.73	14 (70)	6 (30)
III	1 (III 5.1), SD 0.62/ 2 (III 1.6), SD 0.52/ 9 (III 3.2), SD 0/ 18 (III 6.1), SD 0.52/ 20 (III 7.3), SD 0.76/ 21 (III 1.3), SD 0.46/ 22 (III 1.1), SD 0.51/ 24 (III 8.1), SD 0.52/ 28 (III 7.2), SD 0.78/ 31 (III 3.1), SD 0.58/ 33 (III 7.5), SD 0/ 47 (III 1.2), SD 0.49/ 48 (III 2.1), SD 0.50/ 49 (III 1.5), SD 0.83/ 52 (III 4.2), SD 0.52/ 53 (III 1.4), SD 0.41	12 (75)	4 (25)
IV	6 (IV 4.1), SD 0.49/ 11 (IV 5.1), SD 0.46/ 12 (IV 8.1), SD 0/ 13 (IV 7.1), SD 0.60/ 15 (IV 9.2), SD 0.39/ 16 (IV 3.2), SD 0.79/ 25 (IV 6.1), SD 0.53/ 29 (IV 7.2), SD 0.50/ 32 (IV 6.3), SD 0.53/ 34 (IV 2.1), SD 0.53/ 37 (IV 3.1), SD 0.42/ 39 (IV 9.1), SD 0/ 40 (IV 7.3), SD 0/ 44 (IV 6.2), SD 0.82/ 45 (IV 1.1), SD 0.46	13 (86.6)	2 (13.3)

This lower reliability of rating of standards in level I, compared with the other levels, may be explained by the fact that the content of the standards was more open to interpretation. Examples are:

I1.2: The primary healthcare team act as an effective first line of assessment for older people with mental health problems.

I2.2: For people with advanced dementia, the objectives of care encompass improvement in the quality of life throughout the course of the condition, including the terminal phase.

These may be compared with standards from level IV, which was the level that performed most strongly in relation to reliability.

IV8.1: Commissioning staff and agencies have knowledge, experience and expertise in planning mental health services for older people.

IV2.1: Commissioners have an agreed strategy for services for older people with severe and enduring mental health problems.

These standards from level IV were more factual in nature than those in level I.

PART XI

WHAT HAS BEEN LEARNT AND FUTURE DIRECTIONS

CHAPTER 28

Assessment of the Health Advisory Service approach

Robustness of the standards

The Health Advisory Service (HAS) standards to evaluate mental health services for older people were found to have good levels of validity and reliability, as described in Chapters 25 and 26. Compared with other programmes for evaluating health and social care, the development of the methodology was generally more evidence based, as shown in Chapter 22, and comprehensiveness in relation to coverage of the range of mental health services for older people was greater than in other programmes. This was because of the wide range of mechanisms used, and the consistent methodological approach to all aspects of development.

Following literature searches to identify documents to be used for the first draft standards, key people commented on the list of documents, so that this became a definitive list for the client area. The method of content analysis used to extract information from the documents was carefully researched, and the people who carried out the content analysis were trained in the method. The content analysis enabled documented evidence of good practice to be converted into standardised statements.

The mapping process used at the beginning of the standards development identified most aspects of services, and this was added to and refined by the development team. The development team itself was multiprofessional, including representatives not only from all relevant health disciplines, but also from social services, and a carer. This multiprofessional team, in turn, put forward names of individuals and organisations whom it was felt would be appropriate as members of the wider advisory network. Comments on the draft standards, received at the consultative conference, and from postal consultations, were considered and acted on in a consistent way. Discussions with users and carers took the form of focus groups, and the views shared were also written up and processed in a consistent way. The use of focus groups of older people with functional mental illness, and of carers of people with dementia, was in fact a particularly innovative aspect of the standards development. Although some other programmes had consulted users and carers, there was no evidence of such systematic group discussions being held. Learning from pilot reviews, in relation to both the standards document and the review process, was noted and acted on.

With regard to exercises carried out to ascertain the validity of the standards and their reliability in application, the content analysis of the World Health Organization and World Psychiatric Association (1998) consensus statement to check the content validity of the HAS standards used the same methodology as for the content analysis of documents applied earlier in the process, and the people who carried this out had been trained. Following creation by the author of the document for use in the reliability exercise, whereby raters rated extracts from review reports against the standards, a check was carried out by a second person, and it was found that the extracts had been selected accurately.

Although some of the other programmes for evaluating health and social care considered in this book consulted on their standards and methods, there was no evidence in relation to them of consistent mechanisms used to test validity, nor of any reliability testing, as used in developing the HAS standards. The study described here was therefore innovative in having used a robust methodology not only to develop standards, but also to evaluate their validity and reliability.

Comparison with other approaches

Analysis of the various approaches to evaluation of health and social care (*see* Chapter 22) shows how the HAS (from 1997) methodology for evaluation of mental health services for older people compares with the other approaches. With regard to development of the methodology, it compares favourably with other schemes in the soundness of its evidence and consultation base. Like most of the schemes, it used an evidence base in developing standards; it also used an evidence base in developing other aspects of the programme, for example basing its review visits on other similar schemes. It consulted professional organisations in developing both the standards, and other aspects of the programme. These were also consulted on in the development team, and the wider consultative network. Users and carers were consulted in the development of standards, and carers were involved in developing other aspects of the programme, by taking part in pilots.

In relation to features of the programme, HAS's approach had more comprehensive coverage of mental health services for older people than any of the other approaches considered here. Most of the other approaches related to providers only, whereas the HAS approach covered commissioners also. The Social Services Inspectorate (SSI) standards to evaluate mental health services for older people were aimed primarily at those who purchased, registered, inspected or managed services, but covered only residential services.

In terms of evaluating social services in England and Wales, the SSI and the Audit Commission, and the joint reviews undertaken by these two organisations, examined the roles of social services departments as both commissioners and providers of services. However, they included activities relating to all, or many, client groups, and did not focus specifically on mental health services for older people. The same argument may be applied to 'best value', which was a requirement of local authorities generally, rather than of social services departments specifically. The National Care Standards Commission (NCSC) standards, introduced in 2001, although relevant to older people, were not specific to mental health services for older people. Commission for Health Improvement (CHI) reviews of mental health services, at the time of this study, related only to services for adults of working age.

Other approaches which used standards for mental health services for older people included only certain aspects of such services. The Alzheimer's Disease Society (ADS) standards were designed to monitor only those services it provided, and these were for people with Alzheimer's disease or other dementias, thereby excluding services for older people with functional mental illness.

CHAPTER 29

Lessons for the future

Developing standards

As shown in Chapter 27, in the reliability study of the HAS 2000 standards for mental health services for older people, some of the standards that had a standard deviation (SD) higher than the total SD comprised several components, and it would seem that this made it more difficult to rate them consistently. Possible reasons are that a particular site may not provide evidence of all the components, or that raters may differ in the extent to which they consider all the constituent components should be clearly met, in order for the standard to be met. This means that authors of standards need to be aware that, rather than creating such complex standards, it is preferable either to divide such a standard into several standards, or to include some of the constituent parts as criteria, that would need to be met in order for the standard to be met.

An alternative approach would be for the tool devised for use on reviews to contain simpler standards, with or without guidance for the reviewers on how to apply them. This would offer the reviewers more flexibility in the way they used the standards to reach their assessment of services, implying greater reliance on their own knowledge and expertise. However, in HAS 2000 reviews, it was made clear to reviewers that the standards were there to guide them, and were not intended to be used simply as a strict 'checklist'. In addition, it was a deliberate decision on the part of HAS 2000 to apply an evidence-based approach in its reviews, as opposed to that used by HAS prior to 1997, which did not use systematically produced evaluation tools, but did rely instead on the knowledge and expertise of reviewers (*see* Chapter 21).

Some standards included too much material as a result of consultation. This means that actions taken as a result of consultation led to standards that had weaker reliability when applied. This provides a useful pointer for similar exercises carried out in the future. There is currently much emphasis on the role of stakeholders (representatives of professional organisations, royal colleges, voluntary and ethnic minority organisations, users, carers and others) and on consulting them when devising strategies, planning services or, as in this case, developing methodologies. However, although their input is recognised as crucial, the response to their suggestions needs to be a considered one. There is a need to be seen to have consulted widely, and to have taken all stakeholders' views into consideration. However, the process of acting on a plethora of viewpoints in creating verifiable standards is a difficult one.

In some cases, the response to comments may be relatively straightforward, and may involve, for example, simply adding a new standard or additional criteria. A particularly useful example in this regard was where users in the focus groups carried out for this study (*see* Chapter 23) said that they would like more explanation given to them on arrival at a ward, about what would happen during their stay. Where responding to comments involves making changes to existing standards, however, as in the case being discussed here, other factors need to be taken into consideration, such as the reliability of the use of standards. A number of ways of responding to the stakeholders' suggestions need to be considered. As described above, one would be, instead of making the standard longer, using the additional words or phrases suggested by those commenting, to create more than one standard. Another would be to move some of the material into the accompanying criteria. The aim would be to ensure that each standard, and its accompanying criteria, provided the right amount and type of information, so that it could be rated accurately.

A danger here is that the arbitrator, who could be the author or the editor of the standards document, may be biased in the way they make such decisions. They could, for example, decide unilaterally to 'edit out' a valid suggestion from a stakeholder, because they do not personally agree with it. The way round this is to have some kind of 'panel' to ratify decisions made. The editor should list the responses received from stakeholders, and indicate how it is proposed to respond, i.e. the planned changes, and where no changes are envisaged. These should then be discussed with the panel, who should include people from the same categories as the stakeholders consulted. This approach was used by the author, who presented to the development team comments received from consultation, and how it was proposed to respond.

Reliability of the standards in use: the role of the administrator of the standards

As discussed in Chapter 27, the results of the rating exercise, to test the reliability of the use of the HAS 2000 standards for mental health services for older people, showed that the scores for standards in report A had higher SD than those for reports B and C. This may be explained by the fact that part of the methodology used for report A was different from that used for B and C. For B and C, using the document containing the standards and criteria, and the ratings given by the review team, the service development adviser (SDA) completed ratings for each of the criteria for which evidence was available, and the standards were rated accordingly. This completed document was used as the basis for the final report. For report A, although the final report was based on the standards and criteria, the same approach was not used. This has implications for methodologies for evaluating health and social care. It would appear that a consistent system for providing overall ratings for standards (or other comparable 'criteria' for use in measurement) is crucial for a good level of reliability.

For the HAS reviews, the fact that the SDA for report A was different from the SDA for reports B and C was a significant factor in this difference of approach, and demonstrates that the 'administrator' of the method constitutes a facet in the design of the methodology for testing reliability which would merit further consideration. The impact which the 'administrator' has on the application of the standards and the process in a review should be given further thought. Agencies which organise reviews of services often provide training for assessors; however, there is less emphasis on consistent training for those who manage the reviews, in how they do this. Topics that should be covered include how to apply the standards, how to rate them consistently, and the mechanism to be used to provide an overall rating for each standard (or equivalent) in the final report. There may also be scope for training in how to facilitate the review team in order for them to make consistent ratings.

CHAPTER 30

Incentives for improving services

The 'clout' of the evaluating agency

In terms of how seriously the various approaches to evaluating health and social care are taken by the organisations to which they are applied, it may be argued that this would appear to depend on the 'clout' of the agency carrying out the evaluation. As discussed in Chapter 18, in the USA, the Joint Commission on Accreditation of Healthcare Organizations (JCAHO) accreditation system was taken very seriously, because it was granted deemed status, and therefore opened the way for the health providers concerned to receive funding. In Australia, where sanctions could be taken against homes not complying with the standards of the Aged Care Standards and Accreditation Agency (*see* Chapter 18), early indications were that only a small number of providers failed to meet their obligations.

In England (and Wales, in some cases) Commission for Health Improvement (CHI) reviews, SSI inspections, Joint Reviews and Best Value (*see* Chapter 20) were taken seriously by the health organisations and local authorities concerned, not only because these were part of an enforcement process, but also because these evaluation mechanisms, and the agencies which carried them out, had central government backing. Coverage in the media, and anecdotal evidence from those in the health community, bear testimony to the seriousness with which any input from the CHI was treated by the NHS organisations concerned. This was due to the high profile accorded to the CHI by central government, the fact that review findings affected the performance rating of NHS organisations, and to media coverage, of both poor and good performance.

It would follow that, in order for mental health services for older people to improve to be of a universally good standard, there needs to be full commitment to achieving this from central government. Such commitment is much needed. Reviews of mental health services for older people carried out by the HAS established in 1997 showed that, although some parts of services were of a good standard, some remained unacceptable. As described in Chapter 2, services for older people with mental health problems are patchy throughout the country.

The *National Service Framework for Older People*

There may be some grounds for optimism in the *National Service Framework* (NSF) *for Older People* (Department of Health 2001c; Audit Commission 2002) (*see* Chapter 2), which includes a section on mental health. The references show that, like the HAS standards, this NSF is evidence based. The method for devising the framework, like that for the HAS standards, included consultation with a wide range of stakeholders, including experts in the field, service users and carers. The NSF, however, has an advantage over the HAS standards, in that central government requires health organisations and local authorities to follow it. In terms of integration of care, *Better Services for Vulnerable People* (Department of Health 1997) gave clear deadlines by which health and local authorities should have reviewed their assessment processes for older people with complex needs, and their provision of recuperation and rehabilitation services for older people. However, these directives related to older people in general, and did not specifically address the needs of older people with mental health problems.

The NSF has specific milestones, with a deadline. The milestones relating to mental health services for older people touch directly on some of the issues that have been problematic. An integrated mental health service for older people should be included in key joint strategic planning documents. General practitioners (GPs), to whom many older people with mental health problems are likely to turn initially, should have protocols to care for them, and protocols should also be a feature of health and social care systems. The requirement for health and social care systems to have protocols for older people with mental health problems was reinforced by the target in the priorities and planning guidance for 2003–2006 that they should have these in place for care and management by April 2004 (Department of Health 2002b).

Initial assessment of progress on implementation of the NSF, by the Department of Health and commentators, was that some progress had been made, but that it was patchy (Department of Health 2003c; Moore 2003). The CHI, the Audit Commission and the SSI (subsequently, the Commission for Healthcare Audit and Inspection, rebranded the Healthcare Commission, and the Commission for Social Care Inspection) will have responsibility for reviewing progress on implementation (www.chi.nhs.uk). If central government were to accord to this NSF the same high profile that it accorded to the CHI clinical governance reviews (*see* Chapter 20), there would be good prospects for mental health services for older people, in England at least, which were of a universally acceptable standard.

CHAPTER 31

Future research: does evaluation improve care?

As discussed in Chapter 16, organisational evaluations (the type of evaluation focused upon in this book) tend to assess the structure and process of care, whereas clinical and medical evaluations often measure the process and outcome of care. Standards of structure or process are most useful when they are proven to improve care, or if there is a very strong consensus that these are desirable.

The fact that many healthcare organisations in the UK and the other countries considered in this book choose to undergo evaluation of service quality, and that some governments have introduced national evaluation programmes (for example, the CHI and now the Healthcare Commission in the UK) may be considered to constitute a consensus that standards of structure or process are desirable.

In terms of whether such evaluations improve care, we may choose to take the fact that healthcare organisations are using quality assurance mechanisms as an interim or proxy measure for improvements in clinical care and satisfaction for patients and carers. However, there is little or no research or evidence to demonstrate whether the various approaches to evaluating health and social care discussed in this book actually lead to improved care for service users. The lack of a causal link between compliance with standards and improved clinical results has been raised as a problem in relation to accreditation (Shaw and Collins 1995; *see* Chapter 22). The issue has relevance for other evaluation approaches also. Some of the schemes discussed have been in existence for a considerable time (for example, the JCAHO in the USA), giving ample opportunity for such research to have been undertaken.

Studies carried out by the Audit Commission of the impact of its value-for-money studies (*see* Chapter 20) on the NHS showed that implementation of auditors' recommendations was generally disappointing. It was concluded that many factors affected changes in trust activities after a value-for-money audit, including the extent to which the study was in harmony with government and professional thinking, the quality of local auditors' work, and the capacity of local bodies to implement change (Day and Klein 2001). A significant issue in considering both these Audit Commission studies, and the CHI's clinical governance reviews (*see* Chapter 20) is that these evaluations are likely to be most effective when a trust chair or chief executive has an agenda for action, and sees the review report as leverage (Day and Klein 2001, 2002). Indeed, it has been argued that the success or otherwise of any intervention aimed at achieving change in healthcare organisations will depend on the features of the organisation in which it is implemented, and its environment, as well as on the intervention itself (Iles and Sutherland 2001).

The fact remains, however, that substantial resources, which may include the time and energy of staff, stakeholders, users and carers of the organisations being reviewed, staff and reviewers acting on behalf of the reviewing agency, and central government expenditure, are being devoted to formal evaluations of healthcare organisations in a significant number of countries worldwide. In addition, the knowledge that such evaluations are being undertaken is likely to give the impression to many people, including service users, their carers and the general public, that good quality healthcare will result. Research into whether approaches to evaluating health and social care lead to improved care for service users would, therefore, seem to be important, and might include controlled trials of comparable healthcare organisations, some of which do, and some of which do not, use an external quality mechanism, or a study over a period of time of organisations using such mechanisms, to gauge whether, and to what extent, healthcare improves. Great care would naturally need to be taken, to account for other contributory factors.

References

Alzheimer's Disease Society (1996) *The Alzheimer's Disease Society Quality Assurance Initiative.* Alzheimer's Disease Society, London.

Ames D (1997) Geriatric psychiatry in Australia. *International Journal of Geriatric psychiatry.* **12(2)**: 143–4.

Ames D and Flynn E (1994) Dementia services: an Australian view. In: A Burns and R Levy (eds) *Dementia.* Chapman and Hall Medical, London, pp. 611–21.

Arie T (1989) Martin Roth and the 'Psychogeriatricians'. In: K Davison and A Kerr (eds) *Contemporary Themes in Psychiatry – a tribute to Sir Martin Roth.* Gaskell, London, pp. 231–9.

Arie T (1990) Combined geriatrics and psychogeriatrics: a new model. *Geriatric Medicine (20th Anniversary Issue)* April: 24–7.

Arie T and Isaacs AD (1978) The development of psychiatric services for the elderly in Britain. In: F Post and AD Isaacs (eds) *Studies in Geriatric Psychiatry.* John Wiley and Sons, Chichester, pp. 241–61.

Arie T and Jolley D (1982) Making services work: organisation and style of psychogeriatric services. In: R Levy and F Post (eds) *The Psychiatry of Late Life.* Blackwell Scientific, Oxford, pp. 222–51.

Arie T and Jolley D (1998) Psychogeriatric Services. In: R Tallis, H Fillitt and Brocklehurst J (eds) *Brocklehurst's Textbook of Geriatric Medicine and Gerontology* (5e) Churchill Livingstone, Edinburgh, pp. 1567–73.

Atay J, Whitkin M and Manderscheid R (1995) *Data highlights on: utilization of mental health organizations by elderly persons.* Center for Mental Health Services, Rockville, MD.

Audini B, Goddard C, Wattis J *et al.* (2001) *Old Age Psychiatric Day Hospital Survey: final report.* Royal College of Psychiatrists' Research Unit, London.

Audit Commission (1999a) *Making Connections: learning the lessons from joint reviews, 1998/9.* Audit Commission Publications, Abingdon.

Audit Commission (1999b) *A Measure of Success: setting and monitoring local performance targets.* Audit Commission, London.

Audit Commission (2000) *Forget Me Not: mental health services for older people.* Audit Commission, London.

Audit Commission (2002) *Forget Me Not 2002.* Audit Commission, London.

Audit Commission and Department of Health, Social Services Inspectorate (1998) *Getting the Best from Social Services: learning the lessons from Joint Reviews.* Audit Commission Publications, Abingdon.

Bergmann K, Foster EM, Justice AW *et al.* (1978) Management of the demented elderly patient in the community. *British Journal of Psychiatry.* **132**: 441–9.

Bleeker JAC (1994) Dementia services: a continental European view. In: A Burns and R Levy (eds) *Dementia*. Chapman and Hall Medical, London, pp. 581–90.

Bohigas L and Heaton C (2000) Methods for external evaluation of health care institutions. *International Journal for Quality in Health Care.* **12(3)**: 231–8.

Bowie P and Mountain G (1993) Using direct observation to record the behaviour of long-stay patients with dementia. *International Journal of Geriatric Psychiatry.* **8**: 857–64.

Bowling A (1997) *Research Methods in Health: investigating health and health services.* Open University Press, Buckingham and Philadelphia.

British Psychological Society (1995) *Purchasing Clinical Psychology Services: services for older people, their families and other carers. Briefing Paper No. 5.* British Psychological Society, Leicester.

Britton PG and Woods RT (1996) Introduction. In: RT Woods (ed) *Handbook of the Clinical Psychology of Ageing.* John Wiley and Sons, Chichester, pp. 1–19.

Brodaty H and Gresham M (1989) Effect of a training programme to reduce stress in carers of patients with dementia. *BMJ.* **299**: 1375–9.

Brothwood J (1971) The organization and development of services for the aged with special reference to the mentally ill. *British Journal of Psychiatry Special Publication No. 6.* Headley Brothers Ltd, Ashford, pp. 99–112.

Bucht G and Steen B (1990) Development of psychogeriatric medicine in Sweden. *International Psychogeriatrics.* **2(1)**: 73–80.

Canadian Council on Health Services Accreditation (1998a) *Accreditation: step-by-step.* Canadian Council on Health Services Accreditation, Ottowa.

Canadian Council on Health Services Accreditation (1998b) *Council History.* Canadian Council on Health Services Accreditation, Ottowa.

Canadian Council on Health Services Accreditation (1999a) *The Accreditation Standard.* Canadian Council on Health Services Accreditation, Ottowa.

Canadian Council on Health Services Accreditation (1999b) *Fact Sheet.* Canadian Council on Health Services Accreditation, Ottowa.

Canadian Council on Health Services Accreditation (1999c) *Overview of Accreditation.* Canadian Council on Health Services Accreditation, Ottowa.

Carers (Recognition and Services) Act 1995. HMSO, London.

Care Standards Act 2000. The Stationery Office Limited, London.

Care Standards Act 2000: explanatory notes. The Stationery Office Limited, London.

Carmines EG and Zeller RA (1994) Reliability and validity assessment. Part 1. In: MS Lewis-Beck (ed) *Basic Measurement.* Sage Publications, London, Thousand Oaks and New Delhi, pp. 1–58.

Clark P and Bowling A (1989) Observational study of quality of life in NHS nursing homes and a long-stay ward for the elderly. *Ageing and Society.* **9**: 123–48.

Cohen C (1991) Integrated community services. In: J Sadavoy, L Lazarus and L Jarvik (eds) *Comprehensive Review of Geriatric Psychiatry.* American Psychiatric Press, Washington, pp. 613–34.

Commission for Health Improvement (2003a) *Corporate Plan 2003/2004.* Commission for Health Improvement, London.

Commission for Health Improvement (2003b) *Delivering Improvement: annual report 2002/2003*. Commission for Health Improvement, London.

Commonwealth Department of Health and Aged Care: Aged and Community Care (2001) *Two Year Report of Aged Care Reforms: final report and government response*. Department of Health and Aged Care, Australia.

Commonwealth Department of Health and Family Services (1998) *Dementia in Australia*. Australian Government Publishing Service, Canberra.

Commonwealth Department of Health, Housing and Community Services (1991a) *Aged Care Reform Strategy Mid-Term Review 1990–91: progress and directions*. Australian Government Publishing Service, Canberra.

Commonwealth Department of Health, Housing and Community Services (1991b) *Aged Care Reform Strategy Mid-Term Review 1990–91: report*. Australian Government Publishing Service, Canberra.

Congressional Quarterly Inc. (1993), *CQ's Encyclopedia of American Governmental Congress A to Z* (2e). Congressional Quarterly Inc., Washington, DC.

Cooper BA (1997) Principles of service provision in old age psychiatry. In: R Jacoby and C Oppenheimer (eds) *Psychiatry in the Elderly* (2e). Oxford University Press, Oxford, pp. 357–75.

Curlik S, Frazier D and Katz I (1991) Psychiatric aspects of long-term care. In: J Sadovoy, L Lazarus and L Jarvik (eds) *Comprehensive Review of Geriatric Psychiatry*. American Psychiatric Press, Washington, pp. 547–64.

Day P and Klein R (2001) *Auditing the Auditors: audit in the NHS*. The Stationery Office, London.

Day P and Klein R (2002) Who nose best? *Health Service Journal*. **112**(5799): 26–9.

Dean R Briggs K and Lindesay J (1993) The domus philospohy: a prospective evaluation of two residential units for the elderly mentally ill. *International Journal of Geriatric Psychiatry*. **8**: 807–17.

Department of Community Services (1986) *Home and Community Care Program: Commonwealth priorities for service development*. Department of Community Services, Canberra.

Department of Community Services (1986) *Nursing Homes and Hostels Review*. Australian Government Publishing Service, Canberra.

Department of Community Services and Health (1990) *The Problem of Dementia in Australia* (2e). Australian Government Publishing Service, Canberra.

Department of the Environment, Transport and the Regions (1998) *Modern Local Government – in touch with the people*. The Stationery Office, London.

Department of Health, Housing and Community Services (1992) *Putting the Pieces Together: a national action plan for dementia care*. Australian Government Publishing Service, Canberra.

Department of Health, Social Services Inspectorate (1993) *Inspecting for Quality: standards for the residential care of elderly people with mental disorders*. HMSO, London.

Department of Health, Social Services Inspectorate (1996) *At Home with Dementia: inspection of services for older people with dementia in the community*. Department of Health, London.

Department of Health (1997) *Better Services for Vulnerable People* EL(97)62; CI(97)24. Department of Health, London.

Department of Health (1998a) *A First Class Service: quality in the new NHS.* Department of Health, London.

Department of Health (1998b) *Partnership in Action (New Opportunities for Joint Working between Health and Social Services): a discussion document.* Department of Health, London.

Department of Health (1999a) *Effective Care Co-ordination in Mental Health Services: modernising the care programme approach.* Department of Health, London.

Department of Health (1999b) *Fit for the Future? National required standards for residential and nursing homes for older people.* Consultation document. Department of Health, London.

Department of Health, Social Services Inspectorate (2000) *The Social Services Inspectorate: who we are and what we do.* Department of Health, London.

Department of Health (2001a) *Care Homes for Older People: national minimum standards.* The Stationery Office, London.

Department of Health (2001b) *From Vision to Reality.* Department of Health, London.

Department of Health (2001c) *National Service Framework for Older People.* Department of Health, London.

Department of Health (2001d) *Shifting the Balance of Power Within the NHS: securing delivery.* Department of Health, London.

Department of Health (2002a) *Guidance on the Single Assessment Process for Older People.* HSC2002/001; LAC (2002)1. Department of Health, London.

Department of Health (2002b) *Improvement, Expansion and Reform: The next 3 years. Priorities and planning framework 2003–2006.* Department of Health, London.

Department of Health (2003a) *Delivering Investment in General Practice: implementing the new GMS contract.* www.doh.gov.uk/gmscontract/implementation.htm

Department of Health, Social Services Inspectorate (2003b) *Improving Older People's Services: an overview of performance.* Department of Health, London. www.doh.gov.uk/ssi/olderpeople03.htm

Department of Health (2003c) *National Service Framework for Older People: A report of progress and future challenges, 2003.* Department of Health, London.

Department of Health and Social Security (1970a) (Letter dated March 1970). Re: Circular 4/70: *Psycho-Geriatric Assessment Units.* HMSO, London.

Department of Health and Social Security (1970b) *National Health Service Psychogeriatric Assessment Units.* Memorandum with Circular HM(70)11. HMSO, London.

Department of Health and Social Security (1972) *Services for Mental Illness Related to Old Age* HM(72)71. HMSO, London.

Department of Health and Social Security (1975) *Better Services for the Mentally Ill* Cmnd.6233. HMSO, London.

Department of Health and Social Security/Welsh Office (1971) *National Health Service Hospital Advisory Service: Annual Report for 1969–70.* HMSO, London.

Department of National Health and Welfare (1988) *Guidelines for Comprehensive Services to Elderly Persons with Psychiatric Disorders.* Department of National Health and Welfare, Ottawa.

Donabedian A (1980) *Explorations in Quality Assessment and Monotoring. Vol I:*

definition of quality and approaches to its assessment. Health Administration Press, Ann Arbor, Michigan.

Donabedian A (1982) *Explorations in Quality Assessment and Monotoring. Vol II: the criteria and standards of quality.* Health Administration Press, Ann Arbor, Michigan.

Donovan JF, Williams IEI and Wilson TS (1971) A Fully Integrated Psychogeriatric Service. *British Journal of Psychiatry Special Publication No. 6.* Headley Brothers Ltd, Ashford, pp. 113–22.

Duckett SJ (1983) Assuring hospital standards: the introduction of hospital accreditation in Australia. *Australian Journal of Public Administration.* **XLII**: 385–402.

Dunn G (1989) *Design and Analysis of Reliability Studies: the statistical evaluation of measurement errors.* Edward Arnold, London, Melbourne and Auckland.

Dunn G (1992) Design and analysis of reliability studies. *Statistical Methods in Medical Research.* **1**: 123–57.

Dunn G (1997) *The Evaluation of Assessment Errors in Psychology and Education: a self-instructional package for postgraduate students.* School of Epidemiology and Health Sciences, University of Manchester.

Dunn G (1998) Measurement Reliability: A Tutorial for Beginners. Part 1. *The Standard.* Winter 1998. American Society of Quality Control, pp. 23–5.

Easterby-Smith M, Thorpe R and Lowe A (1991) *Management Research: an introduction.* Sage Publications, London.

Estes CL (1995) Mental health services for the elderly: key policy elements. In: M Gatz (ed) *Emerging Issues in Mental Health and Aging.* American Psychological Association, Washington DC, pp. 303–27.

Fasey C (1994) The day hospital in old age psychiatry: the case against. *International Journal of Geriatric Psychiatry.* **9**: 519–23.

Finch J and Orrell M (1999) Involving users and carers in developing standards for mental health services for older people. *Managing Community Care.* **7(6)**: 25–9.

Gatz M and Finkel SI (1995) Education and Training of Mental Health Service Providers. In: M Gatz (ed) *Emerging Issues in Mental Health and Aging.* American Psychological Association, Washington DC, pp. 282–302.

Goetschalckx C (1997) *European Transitional Alzheimer's Study: National Report - Luxembourg.* Association Luxembourg Alzheimer, Luxembourg.

Health Act 1999. The Stationery Office, London.

Health Advisory Service 2000 (1999) *Standards for Mental Health Services for Older People.* Pavilion Publishing Ltd, Brighton.

Healthbeat (January 2000). McCrone Publications Inc., Edmonton, Alberta.

Health Quality Service (1999) *The Work of the Health Quality Service.* Health Quality Service, London.

Heidemann EG (2000) Moving to global standards for accreditation processes: the ExPeRT Project in a larger context. *International Journal for Quality in Health Care* **12(3)**: 227–30

Higginson I (1994) Quality of care and evaluating services. *International Review of Psychiatry.* **6**: 5–14.

Hospital Accreditation Programme (2000) *Annual Report April 1999–March 2000.* CASPE Research, London.

Howard R (1994) Day hospitals: the case in favour. *International Journal of Geriatric Psychiatry.* **9**: 525–9.

Howe AL (1997) From states of confusion to a national action plan for dementia care: the development of policies for dementia care in Australia. *International Journal of Geriatric Psychiatry.* **12(2)**: 165–71.

Human Rights and Equal Opportunities Commission (1993) *Human Rights and Mental Illness: report of the national inquiry into the human rights of people with mental illness.* Australian Government Publishing Service, Canberra.

Iles V and Sutherland K (2001) *Organisational Change: a review for health care managers, professionals and researchers.* National Co-ordinating Centre for NHS Service Delivery and Organisation R&D, London School of Hygiene and Tropical Medicine, London.

Joint Commission on Accreditation of Healthcare Organizations (1997) *Long Term Care: survey and accreditation process guide.* Joint Commission on Accreditation of Healthcare Organizations, Illinois.

Jolley D and Arie T (1978) The organisation of psychogeriatric services. *British Journal of Psychiatry.* **132**: 1–11.

Jolley D and Arie T (1992) Developments in psychogeriatric services. In: T Arie (ed) *Recent Advances in Psychogeriatrics No. 2.* Churchill Livingstone, Edinburgh, pp. 117–135.

Kay DWK, Roth M and Hall MRP (1966) Special problems of the aged and the organization of hospital services. *British Medical Journal.* **2**: 967–72.

Klazinga N (2000) Re-engineering trust: the adoption and adaption of four models for external quality assurance of health care services in western European health care systems. *International Journal for Quality in Health Care.* **12(3)**: 183–9.

Knight BG and Kaskie B (1995) Models for mental health service delivery to older adults. In: M Gatz (ed) *Emerging Issues in Mental Health and Aging.* American Psychological Association, Washington DC, pp. 231–55.

Knight BG, Rickards L, Rabins P *et al.* (1995) Community-based services for mentally ill people. In: B Knight, L Teri, P Wohlford and J Santos (eds) *Mental Health Services for Older Adults: implications for training and practice.* American Psychological Association, Washington, DC.

Knight BG, Woods B, Kaskie B *et al.* (1998) Community mental health services in the United States and the United Kingdom: a comparative systems approach. In: AS Bellack and M Herson (eds) *Comprehensive Clinical Psychology. Volume 7.* Elsevier, Oxford.

Koenig HG, George LK and Schneider R (1994) Mental health care for older adults in the year 2000: a dangerous and avoided topic. *The Gerontologist.* **34(5)**: 674–9.

Lindesay J, Briggs K, Lawes M *et al.* (1991) The domus philosophy: a comparative evaluation of a new approach to residential care for the demented elderly. *International Journal of Geriatric Psychiatry.* **6**: 727–36.

Mace N and Rabins P (1984) *A Survey of Day Care for the Demented Adult in the United States.* National Council on the Aging, Inc, Washington DC.

MacMillan D (1960) Preventive geriatrics: opportunities of a community mental health service. *The Lancet.* **ii**: 1439–40.

Mental Health Services in Alberta (1999) *Healthbeat.* **2(4)**: 1–2. McCrone Publications Inc, Edmonton.

Moore A (2003) Age concerns. *Health Service Journal.* **113(5848)**: 37–38, 41.

Nabitz U, Klazinga N and Walburg J (2000) The EFQM excellence model: European and Dutch experiences with the EFQM approach in health care. *International Journal for Quality in Health Care.* **12(3)**: 191–201.

National Association of Health Authorities (1988) *Towards Good Practice in Small Hospitals.*

National Health Service (1972) *Annual Report of the Hospital Advisory Service to the Secretary of State for Social Services and Secretary of State for Wales for the Year 1971.* HMSO, London.

National Health Service (1975; 2nd impression, 1976) *Annual Report of the Hospital Advisory Service to the Secretary of State for Social Services and Secretary of State for Wales for the Year 1974.* HMSO, London.

National Health Service (1976) *Annual Report of the Hospital Advisory Service to the Secretary of State for Social Services and Secretary of State for Wales for the Year 1975.* HMSO, London.

NHS Health Advisory Service (1982) *The Rising Tide: developing services for mental illness in old age.* NHS Health Advisory Service, Sutton, Surrey.

NHS Health Advisory Service (1985) *Annual Report (June 1984–June 1985).* NHS Health Advisory Service, Sutton, Surrey.

NHS Health Advisory Service (1996) *Making a Mark: the annual report of the director for 1994–95.* HMSO, London.

National Health Service Reform and Health Care Professions Act 2002. The Stationery Office Limited, London.

New South Wales Ministerial Implementation Committee on Mental Health and Developmental Disability (1988) *Report to the Minister for Health, Psychogeriatrics Working Party: Volume 3.*

Nijkamp P, Pacolet J, Spinnewyn H *et al.* (1991) *Services for the Elderly in Europe: a cross-national comparative study (2e).* Katholieke Universiteit Leuven; Vrije Universiteit Amsterdam, Leuven.

Office of the Deputy Prime Minister (2001) *Strong Local Leadership: quality public services.* Office of the Deputy Prime Minister, London.

Office of the Federal Register National Archives and Records Administration (1999) *The United States Government Manual 1999–2000.* US Government Printing Office, Washington, DC.

Parliament of the Commonwealth of Australia (1982) *In a Home or at Home: accommodation and home care for the aged.* Australian Government Publishing Services, Canberra.

Pearsall J (ed) (1998; thumb index edition, 1999) *New Oxford Dictionary of English.* Oxford University Press, Oxford.

Registered Homes Act (1984) HMSO, London.

Reifler BV (1997) The practice of geriatric psychiatry in three countries: observations of an American in the British Isles. *International Journal of Geriatric Psychiatry.* **12**: 795–807.

Reifler BV and Cohen W (1998) Practice of geriatric psychiatry and mental health services for the elderly: results of an international survey. *International Psychogeriatrics.* **10(4)**: 351–7.

Richardson B and Orrell M (2002) Home assessments in old age psychiatry. *Advances in Psychiatric Treatment.* **8**: 59–65.

Robinson RA (1962) The practice of a psychiatric geriatric unit. *Gerontologica Clinica.* **1**: 1–19.

Rosen AL, Pancake JA and Rickards L (1995) Mental health policy and older Americans: historical and current perspectives. In: M Gatz (ed) *Emerging Issues in Mental Health and Aging.* American Psychological Association, Washington DC, pp. 1–18.

Royal College of Physicians and Royal College of Psychiatrists (1989) *Care of Elderly People with Mental Illness: specialist services and training.* Royal College of Physicians and Royal College of Psychiatrists, London.

Royal College of Psychiatrists' Research Unit (1996, unpublished) *Standards for Mental Health Services Organisations: source book.* Royal College of Psychiatrists' Research Unit, London.

Royal College of Psychiatrists and Royal College of Physicians (1998) *The Care of Older People with Mental Illness: specialist services and medical training: report of a joint working party of the Royal College of Psychiatrists and Royal College of Physicians.* Council Report CR69. Royal College of Psychiatrists and Royal College of Physicians, London.

Schyve PM (2000) The evolution of external quality evaluation: observations from the Joint Commission on Accreditation of Healthcare Organizations. *International Journal for Quality in Health Care.* **12(3)**: 255–8.

Scrivens E (1995a) *Accreditation: protecting the professional or the consumer?* Open University Press, Buckingham and Philadelphia.

Scrivens E (1995b) International trends in accreditation. *International Journal of Health Planning and Management* **10**: 165–81.

Scrivens EJ, Klein R and Steiner A (1995) Accreditation: what can we learn from the Anglophone model? *Health Policy.* **34**: 193–204.

Secretary of State for Health (1997) *The New NHS: modern – dependable.* The Stationery Office, London.

Secretary of State for Health (1998) *Modernising Social Services.* The Stationery Office, London.

Secretary of State for Health (2000) *The NHS Plan: a plan for investment, a plan for reform.* The Stationery Office, London.

Secretary of State for Health (2002) *Delivering the NHS Plan: next steps on investment; next steps on reform.* The Stationery Office, Norwich.

Secretaries of State for Health, Social Security, Wales and Scotland (1989) *Caring for People: community care in the next decade and beyond.* HMSO, London.

Secretaries of State for Health, Wales, Northern Ireland and Scotland (1989) *Working for Patients.* HMSO, London.

Secretary of State for Social Services, Secretary of State for Scotland, Secretary of State for Wales and Secretary of State for Northern Ireland (1981) *Growing Older.* Cmnd 8173. HMSO, London.

Shavelson RJ and Webb NM (1991) *Generalizability Theory: a primer.* Sage Publications, California, London and New Delhi.

Shaw CD (1982) Monitoring and standards in the NHS: (2) standards. *British Medical Journal.* **284**: 288–9.

Shaw CD (1997) Accreditation Standards in Europe. *Journal d'Economie Médicale.* **T.15, No.6:** 411–17.

Shaw CD (2000) External quality mechanisms for health care: summary of the ExPeRT project on *visitatie,* accreditation, EFQM and ISO assessment in European Union countries. *International Journal for Quality in Health Care.* **12(3):** 169–75.

Shaw CD and Brooks TE (1991) Health Service accreditation in the United Kingdom. *Quality Assurance in Health Care.* **3(3):** 133–40.

Shaw CD and Collins CD (1995) Health service accreditation: report of a pilot programme for community hospitals. *British Medical Journal.* **310:** 781–4.

Shulman K (1981) Service Innovations in Geriatric Psychiatry. In: T Arie (ed) *Health Care of the Elderly: essays in old age medicine, psychiatry and services.* Croom Helm, London, pp. 214–23.

Shulman K and Arie T (1991) UK survey of psychiatric services for the elderly: direction for developing services. *Canadian Journal of Psychiatry.* **36:** 169–75.

Snowdon J (1987) Psychiatric services for the elderly. *Australian and New Zealand Journal of Psychiatry.* **21:** 131–6.

Social Security Administration (1996) *Social Security: understanding the benefits.* Social Security Administration, USA.

Social Security Administration (1999) *Annual Statistical Supplement 1999 to the Social Security Bulletin.* Social Security Administration, Washington, DC.

Spencer G and Jolley D (1999) Planning services for the elderly. *Advances in Psychiatric Treatment.* **5:** 202–12.

Vidall S-A (1998) King's Fund Organisational Audit: more ticks than boxes. *Journal of Quality in Clinical Practice.* **18:** 83–8.

Weissart WG, Elston JM, Bolda EJ *et al.* (1989) Models of adult care: findings from a national survey. *Gerontologist.* **29:** 640–9.

Wing J, Rix S and Curtis R (1995) *Clinical Standards Advisory Group: Schizophrenia. Volume 2. Protocol for Assessing People with Severe Mental Illness.* HMSO, London.

World Health Organization Division of Mental Health and Prevention of Substance Abuse (1997) *Quality Assurance in Mental Health Care: check-lists and glossaries. Volume 2.* World Health Organization.

World Health Organization Regional Office for Europe (1979) Psychogeriatric Care in the Community. *Public Health in Europe. No 10.* World Health Organization, Copenhagen.

World Health Organization and World Psychiatric Association (1998) Organization of care in psychiatry of the elderly – a technical consensus statement. *Aging and Mental Health.* **2(3):** 246–52.

www.chi.nhs.uk

www.doh.gov.uk

www.ratings.chi.nhs.uk

Zarit SH and Zarit JM (1998) *Mental Disorders in Older Adults: fundamentals of assessment and treatment.* The Guildford Press, New York.

Zisselman M and Rovner BW (1994) North American services for patients with dementia. In: A Burns and R Levy (eds) *Dementia.* Chapman and Hall Medical, London, pp. 591–9.

Index